Orthopaedic Technologist Certified Exam

SECRETS

Study Guide

Your Key to Exam Success

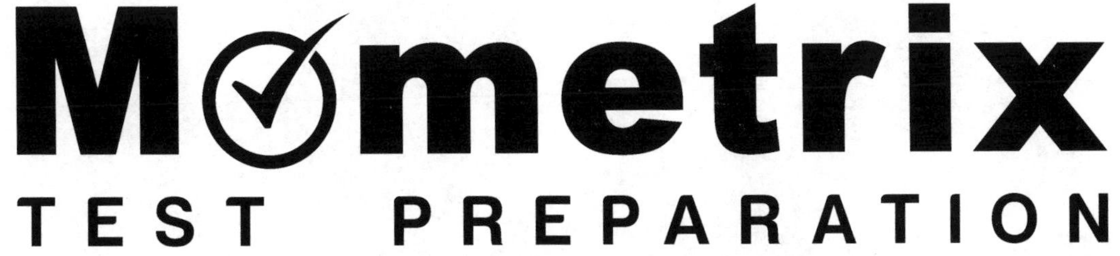

DEAR FUTURE EXAM SUCCESS STORY

First of all, **THANK YOU** for purchasing Mometrix study materials!

Second, congratulations! You are one of the few determined test-takers who are committed to doing whatever it takes to excel on your exam. **You have come to the right place.** We developed these study materials with one goal in mind: to deliver you the information you need in a format that's concise and easy to use.

In addition to optimizing your guide for the content of the test, we've outlined our recommended steps for breaking down the preparation process into small, attainable goals so you can make sure you stay on track.

We've also analyzed the entire test-taking process, identifying the most common pitfalls and showing how you can overcome them and be ready for any curveball the test throws you.

Standardized testing is one of the biggest obstacles on your road to success, which only increases the importance of doing well in the high-pressure, high-stakes environment of test day. Your results on this test could have a significant impact on your future, and this guide provides the information and practical advice to help you achieve your full potential on test day.

Your success is our success

We would love to hear from you! If you would like to share the story of your exam success or if you have any questions or comments in regard to our products, please contact us at **800-673-8175** or **support@mometrix.com**.

Thanks again for your business and we wish you continued success!

Sincerely,
The Mometrix Test Preparation Team

Need more help? Check out our flashcards at:
http://MometrixFlashcards.com/OrthopaedicTech

Written and edited by the Mometrix Exam Secrets Test Prep Team
Printed in the United States of America

TABLE OF CONTENTS

Introduction

Thank you for purchasing this resource! You have made the choice to prepare yourself for a test that could have a huge impact on your future, and this guide is designed to help you be fully ready for test day. Obviously, it's important to have a solid understanding of the test material, but you also need to be prepared for the unique environment and stressors of the test, so that you can perform to the best of your abilities.

For this purpose, the first section that appears in this guide is the **Secret Keys**. We've devoted countless hours to meticulously researching what works and what doesn't, and we've boiled down our findings to the five most impactful steps you can take to improve your performance on the test. We start at the beginning with study planning and move through the preparation process, all the way to the testing strategies that will help you get the most out of what you know when you're finally sitting in front of the test.

We recommend that you start preparing for your test as far in advance as possible. However, if you've bought this guide as a last-minute study resource and only have a few days before your test, we recommend that you skip over the first two Secret Keys since they address a long-term study plan.

If you struggle with **test anxiety**, we strongly encourage you to check out our recommendations for how you can overcome it. Test anxiety is a formidable foe, but it can be beaten, and we want to make sure you have the tools you need to defeat it.

Secret Key #1 – Plan Big, Study Small

There's a lot riding on your performance. If you want to ace this test, you're going to need to keep your skills sharp and the material fresh in your mind. You need a plan that lets you review everything you need to know while still fitting in your schedule. We'll break this strategy down into three categories.

Information Organization

Start with the information you already have: the official test outline. From this, you can make a complete list of all the concepts you need to cover before the test. Organize these concepts into groups that can be studied together, and create a list of any related vocabulary you need to learn so you can brush up on any difficult terms. You'll want to keep this vocabulary list handy once you actually start studying since you may need to add to it along the way.

Time Management

Once you have your set of study concepts, decide how to spread them out over the time you have left before the test. Break your study plan into small, clear goals so you have a manageable task for each day and know exactly what you're doing. Then just focus on one small step at a time. When you manage your time this way, you don't need to spend hours at a time studying. Studying a small block of content for a short period each day helps you retain information better and avoid stressing over how much you have left to do. You can relax knowing that you have a plan to cover everything in time. In order for this strategy to be effective though, you have to start studying early and stick to your schedule. Avoid the exhaustion and futility that comes from last-minute cramming!

Study Environment

The environment you study in has a big impact on your learning. Studying in a coffee shop, while probably more enjoyable, is not likely to be as fruitful as studying in a quiet room. It's important to keep distractions to a minimum. You're only planning to study for a short block of time, so make the most of it. Don't pause to check your phone or get up to find a snack. It's also important to **avoid multitasking**. Research has consistently shown that multitasking will make your studying dramatically less effective. Your study area should also be comfortable and well-lit so you don't have the distraction of straining your eyes or sitting on an uncomfortable chair.

The time of day you study is also important. You want to be rested and alert. Don't wait until just before bedtime. Study when you'll be most likely to comprehend and remember. Even better, if you know what time of day your test will be, set that time aside for study. That way your brain will be used to working on that subject at that specific time and you'll have a better chance of recalling information.

Finally, it can be helpful to team up with others who are studying for the same test. Your actual studying should be done in as isolated an environment as possible, but the work of organizing the information and setting up the study plan can be divided up. In between study sessions, you can discuss with your teammates the concepts that you're all studying and quiz each other on the details. Just be sure that your teammates are as serious about the test as you are. If you find that your study time is being replaced with social time, you might need to find a new team.

Secret Key #2 – Make Your Studying Count

You're devoting a lot of time and effort to preparing for this test, so you want to be absolutely certain it will pay off. This means doing more than just reading the content and hoping you can remember it on test day. It's important to make every minute of study count. There are two main areas you can focus on to make your studying count:

Retention

It doesn't matter how much time you study if you can't remember the material. You need to make sure you are retaining the concepts. To check your retention of the information you're learning, try recalling it at later times with minimal prompting. Try carrying around flashcards and glance at one or two from time to time or ask a friend who's also studying for the test to quiz you.

To enhance your retention, look for ways to put the information into practice so that you can apply it rather than simply recalling it. If you're using the information in practical ways, it will be much easier to remember. Similarly, it helps to solidify a concept in your mind if you're not only reading it to yourself but also explaining it to someone else. Ask a friend to let you teach them about a concept you're a little shaky on (or speak aloud to an imaginary audience if necessary). As you try to summarize, define, give examples, and answer your friend's questions, you'll understand the concepts better and they will stay with you longer. Finally, step back for a big picture view and ask yourself how each piece of information fits with the whole subject. When you link the different concepts together and see them working together as a whole, it's easier to remember the individual components.

Finally, practice showing your work on any multi-step problems, even if you're just studying. Writing out each step you take to solve a problem will help solidify the process in your mind, and you'll be more likely to remember it during the test.

Modality

Modality simply refers to the means or method by which you study. Choosing a study modality that fits your own individual learning style is crucial. No two people learn best in exactly the same way, so it's important to know your strengths and use them to your advantage.

For example, if you learn best by visualization, focus on visualizing a concept in your mind and draw an image or a diagram. Try color-coding your notes, illustrating them, or creating symbols that will trigger your mind to recall a learned concept. If you learn best by hearing or discussing information, find a study partner who learns the same way or read aloud to yourself. Think about how to put the information in your own words. Imagine that you are giving a lecture on the topic and record yourself so you can listen to it later.

For any learning style, flashcards can be helpful. Organize the information so you can take advantage of spare moments to review. Underline key words or phrases. Use different colors for different categories. Mnemonic devices (such as creating a short list in which every item starts with the same letter) can also help with retention. Find what works best for you and use it to store the information in your mind most effectively and easily.

Secret Key #3 – Practice the Right Way

Your success on test day depends not only on how many hours you put into preparing, but also on whether you prepared the right way. It's good to check along the way to see if your studying is paying off. One of the most effective ways to do this is by taking practice tests to evaluate your progress. Practice tests are useful because they show exactly where you need to improve. Every time you take a practice test, pay special attention to these three groups of questions:

- The questions you got wrong
- The questions you had to guess on, even if you guessed right
- The questions you found difficult or slow to work through

This will show you exactly what your weak areas are, and where you need to devote more study time. Ask yourself why each of these questions gave you trouble. Was it because you didn't understand the material? Was it because you didn't remember the vocabulary? Do you need more repetitions on this type of question to build speed and confidence? Dig into those questions and figure out how you can strengthen your weak areas as you go back to review the material.

Additionally, many practice tests have a section explaining the answer choices. It can be tempting to read the explanation and think that you now have a good understanding of the concept. However, an explanation likely only covers part of the question's broader context. Even if the explanation makes sense, **go back and investigate** every concept related to the question until you're positive you have a thorough understanding.

As you go along, keep in mind that the practice test is just that: practice. Memorizing these questions and answers will not be very helpful on the actual test because it is unlikely to have any of the same exact questions. If you only know the right answers to the sample questions, you won't be prepared for the real thing. **Study the concepts** until you understand them fully, and then you'll be able to answer any question that shows up on the test.

It's important to wait on the practice tests until you're ready. If you take a test on your first day of study, you may be overwhelmed by the amount of material covered and how much you need to learn. Work up to it gradually.

On test day, you'll need to be prepared for answering questions, managing your time, and using the test-taking strategies you've learned. It's a lot to balance, like a mental marathon that will have a big impact on your future. Like training for a marathon, you'll need to start slowly and work your way up. When test day arrives, you'll be ready.

Start with the strategies you've read in the first two Secret Keys—plan your course and study in the way that works best for you. If you have time, consider using multiple study resources to get different approaches to the same concepts. It can be helpful to see difficult concepts from more than one angle. Then find a good source for practice tests. Many times, the test website will suggest potential study resources or provide sample tests.

Practice Test Strategy

If you're able to find at least three practice tests, we recommend this strategy:

1. Take the first test with no time constraints and with your notes and study guide handy. Take your time and focus on applying the strategies you've learned.
2. Take the second practice test open-book as well, but set a timer and practice pacing yourself to finish in time.
3. Take any other practice tests as if it were test day. Set a timer and put away your study materials. Sit at a table or desk in a quiet room, imagine yourself at the testing center, and answer questions as quickly and accurately as possible.
4. Keep repeating step 3 on a regular basis until you run out of practice tests or it's time for the actual test. Your mind will be ready for the schedule and stress of test day, and you'll be able to focus on recalling the material you've learned.

Secret Key #4 – Pace Yourself

Once you're fully prepared for the material on the test, your biggest challenge on test day will be managing your time. Just knowing that the clock is ticking can make you panic even if you have plenty of time left. Work on pacing yourself so you can build confidence against the time constraints of the exam. Pacing is a difficult skill to master, especially in a high-pressure environment, so **practice is vital**.

Set time expectations for your pace based on how much time is available. For example, if a section has 60 questions and the time limit is 30 minutes, you know you have to average 30 seconds or less per question in order to answer them all. Although 30 seconds is the hard limit, set 25 seconds per question as your goal, so you reserve extra time to spend on harder questions. When you budget extra time for the harder questions, you no longer have any reason to stress when those questions take longer to answer.

Don't let this time expectation distract you from working through the test at a calm, steady pace, but keep it in mind so you don't spend too much time on any one question. Recognize that taking extra time on one question you don't understand may keep you from answering two that you do understand later in the test. If your time limit for a question is up and you're still not sure of the answer, mark it and move on, and come back to it later if the time and the test format allow. If the testing format doesn't allow you to return to earlier questions, just make an educated guess; then put it out of your mind and move on.

On the easier questions, be careful not to rush. It may seem wise to hurry through them so you have more time for the challenging ones, but it's not worth missing one if you know the concept and just didn't take the time to read the question fully. Work efficiently but make sure you understand the question and have looked at all of the answer choices, since more than one may seem right at first.

Even if you're paying attention to the time, you may find yourself a little behind at some point. You should speed up to get back on track, but do so wisely. Don't panic; just take a few seconds less on each question until you're caught up. Don't guess without thinking, but do look through the answer choices and eliminate any you know are wrong. If you can get down to two choices, it is often worthwhile to guess from those. Once you've chosen an answer, move on and don't dwell on any that you skipped or had to hurry through. If a question was taking too long, chances are it was one of the harder ones, so you weren't as likely to get it right anyway.

On the other hand, if you find yourself getting ahead of schedule, it may be beneficial to slow down a little. The more quickly you work, the more likely you are to make a careless mistake that will affect your score. You've budgeted time for each question, so don't be afraid to spend that time. Practice an efficient but careful pace to get the most out of the time you have.

Secret Key #5 – Have a Plan for Guessing

When you're taking the test, you may find yourself stuck on a question. Some of the answer choices seem better than others, but you don't see the one answer choice that is obviously correct. What do you do?

The scenario described above is very common, yet most test takers have not effectively prepared for it. Developing and practicing a plan for guessing may be one of the single most effective uses of your time as you get ready for the exam.

In developing your plan for guessing, there are three questions to address:

- When should you start the guessing process?
- How should you narrow down the choices?
- Which answer should you choose?

When to Start the Guessing Process

Unless your plan for guessing is to select C every time (which, despite its merits, is not what we recommend), you need to leave yourself enough time to apply your answer elimination strategies. Since you have a limited amount of time for each question, that means that if you're going to give yourself the best shot at guessing correctly, you have to decide quickly whether or not you will guess.

Of course, the best-case scenario is that you don't have to guess at all, so first, see if you can answer the question based on your knowledge of the subject and basic reasoning skills. Focus on the key words in the question and try to jog your memory of related topics. Give yourself a chance to bring the knowledge to mind, but once you realize that you don't have (or you can't access) the knowledge you need to answer the question, it's time to start the guessing process.

It's almost always better to start the guessing process too early than too late. It only takes a few seconds to remember something and answer the question from knowledge. Carefully eliminating wrong answer choices takes longer. Plus, going through the process of eliminating answer choices can actually help jog your memory.

Summary: Start the guessing process as soon as you decide that you can't answer the question based on your knowledge.

How to Narrow Down the Choices

The next chapter in this book (**Test-Taking Strategies**) includes a wide range of strategies for how to approach questions and how to look for answer choices to eliminate. You will definitely want to read those carefully, practice them, and figure out which ones work best for you. Here though, we're going to address a mindset rather than a particular strategy.

Your chances of guessing an answer correctly depend on how many options you are choosing from.

How many choices you have	How likely you are to guess correctly
5	20%
4	25%
3	33%
2	50%
1	100%

You can see from this chart just how valuable it is to be able to eliminate incorrect answers and make an educated guess, but there are two things that many test takers do that cause them to miss out on the benefits of guessing:

- Accidentally eliminating the correct answer
- Selecting an answer based on an impression

We'll look at the first one here, and the second one in the next section.

To avoid accidentally eliminating the correct answer, we recommend a thought exercise called **the $5 challenge**. In this challenge, you only eliminate an answer choice from contention if you are willing to bet $5 on it being wrong. Why $5? Five dollars is a small but not insignificant amount of money. It's an amount you could afford to lose but wouldn't want to throw away. And while losing $5 once might not hurt too much, doing it twenty times will set you back $100. In the same way, each small decision you make—eliminating a choice here, guessing on a question there—won't by itself impact your score very much, but when you put them all together, they can make a big difference. By holding each answer choice elimination decision to a higher standard, you can reduce the risk of accidentally eliminating the correct answer.

The $5 challenge can also be applied in a positive sense: If you are willing to bet $5 that an answer choice *is* correct, go ahead and mark it as correct.

Summary: Only eliminate an answer choice if you are willing to bet $5 that it is wrong.

Which Answer to Choose

You're taking the test. You've run into a hard question and decided you'll have to guess. You've eliminated all the answer choices you're willing to bet $5 on. Now you have to pick an answer. Why do we even need to talk about this? Why can't you just pick whichever one you feel like when the time comes?

The answer to these questions is that if you don't come into the test with a plan, you'll rely on your impression to select an answer choice, and if you do that, you risk falling into a trap. The test writers know that everyone who takes their test will be guessing on some of the questions, so they intentionally write wrong answer choices to seem plausible. You still have to pick an answer though, and if the wrong answer choices are designed to look right, how can you ever be sure that you're not falling for their trap? The best solution we've found to this dilemma is to take the decision out of your hands entirely. Here is the process we recommend:

Once you've eliminated any choices that you are confident (willing to bet $5) are wrong, select the first remaining choice as your answer.

Whether you choose to select the first remaining choice, the second, or the last, the important thing is that you use some preselected standard. Using this approach guarantees that you will not be enticed into selecting an answer choice that looks right, because you are not basing your decision on how the answer choices look.

This is not meant to make you question your knowledge. Instead, it is to help you recognize the difference between your knowledge and your impressions. There's a huge difference between thinking an answer is right because of what you know, and thinking an answer is right because it looks or sounds like it should be right.

Summary: To ensure that your selection is appropriately random, make a predetermined selection from among all answer choices you have not eliminated.

Test-Taking Strategies

This section contains a list of test-taking strategies that you may find helpful as you work through the test. By taking what you know and applying logical thought, you can maximize your chances of answering any question correctly!

It is very important to realize that every question is different and every person is different: no single strategy will work on every question, and no single strategy will work for every person. That's why we've included all of them here, so you can try them out and determine which ones work best for different types of questions and which ones work best for you.

Question Strategies

Read Carefully

Read the question and answer choices carefully. Don't miss the question because you misread the terms. You have plenty of time to read each question thoroughly and make sure you understand what is being asked. Yet a happy medium must be attained, so don't waste too much time. You must read carefully, but efficiently.

Contextual Clues

Look for contextual clues. If the question includes a word you are not familiar with, look at the immediate context for some indication of what the word might mean. Contextual clues can often give you all the information you need to decipher the meaning of an unfamiliar word. Even if you can't determine the meaning, you may be able to narrow down the possibilities enough to make a solid guess at the answer to the question.

Prefixes

If you're having trouble with a word in the question or answer choices, try dissecting it. Take advantage of every clue that the word might include. Prefixes and suffixes can be a huge help. Usually they allow you to determine a basic meaning. Pre- means before, post- means after, pro - is positive, de- is negative. From prefixes and suffixes, you can get an idea of the general meaning of the word and try to put it into context.

Hedge Words

Watch out for critical hedge words, such as *likely, may, can, sometimes, often, almost, mostly, usually, generally, rarely,* and *sometimes.* Question writers insert these hedge phrases to cover every possibility. Often an answer choice will be wrong simply because it leaves no room for exception. Be on guard for answer choices that have definitive words such as *exactly* and *always.*

Switchback Words

Stay alert for *switchbacks.* These are the words and phrases frequently used to alert you to shifts in thought. The most common switchback words are *but, although,* and *however.* Others include *nevertheless, on the other hand, even though, while, in spite of, despite, regardless of.* Switchback words are important to catch because they can change the direction of the question or an answer choice.

Face Value

When in doubt, use common sense. Accept the situation in the problem at face value. Don't read too much into it. These problems will not require you to make wild assumptions. If you have to go beyond creativity and warp time or space in order to have an answer choice fit the question, then you should move on and consider the other answer choices. These are normal problems rooted in reality. The applicable relationship or explanation may not be readily apparent, but it is there for you to figure out. Use your common sense to interpret anything that isn't clear.

Answer Choice Strategies

Answer Selection

The most thorough way to pick an answer choice is to identify and eliminate wrong answers until only one is left, then confirm it is the correct answer. Sometimes an answer choice may immediately seem right, but be careful. The test writers will usually put more than one reasonable answer choice on each question, so take a second to read all of them and make sure that the other choices are not equally obvious. As long as you have time left, it is better to read every answer choice than to pick the first one that looks right without checking the others.

Answer Choice Families

An answer choice family consists of two (in rare cases, three) answer choices that are very similar in construction and cannot all be true at the same time. If you see two answer choices that are direct opposites or parallels, one of them is usually the correct answer. For instance, if one answer choice says that quantity *x* increases and another either says that quantity *x* decreases (opposite) or says that quantity *y* increases (parallel), then those answer choices would fall into the same family. An answer choice that doesn't match the construction of the answer choice family is more likely to be incorrect. Most questions will not have answer choice families, but when they do appear, you should be prepared to recognize them.

Eliminate Answers

Eliminate answer choices as soon as you realize they are wrong, but make sure you consider all possibilities. If you are eliminating answer choices and realize that the last one you are left with is also wrong, don't panic. Start over and consider each choice again. There may be something you missed the first time that you will realize on the second pass.

Avoid Fact Traps

Don't be distracted by an answer choice that is factually true but doesn't answer the question. You are looking for the choice that answers the question. Stay focused on what the question is asking for so you don't accidentally pick an answer that is true but incorrect. Always go back to the question and make sure the answer choice you've selected actually answers the question and is not merely a true statement.

Extreme Statements

In general, you should avoid answers that put forth extreme actions as standard practice or proclaim controversial ideas as established fact. An answer choice that states the "process should be used in certain situations, if..." is much more likely to be correct than one that states the "process should be discontinued completely." The first is a calm rational statement and doesn't even make a definitive, uncompromising stance, using a hedge word *if* to provide wiggle room, whereas the second choice is a radical idea and far more extreme.

Benchmark

As you read through the answer choices and you come across one that seems to answer the question well, mentally select that answer choice. This is not your final answer, but it's the one that will help you evaluate the other answer choices. The one that you selected is your benchmark or standard for judging each of the other answer choices. Every other answer choice must be compared to your benchmark. That choice is correct until proven otherwise by another answer choice beating it. If you find a better answer, then that one becomes your new benchmark. Once you've decided that no other choice answers the question as well as your benchmark, you have your final answer.

Predict the Answer

Before you even start looking at the answer choices, it is often best to try to predict the answer. When you come up with the answer on your own, it is easier to avoid distractions and traps because you will know exactly what to look for. The right answer choice is unlikely to be word-for-word what you came up with, but it should be a close match. Even if you are confident that you have the right answer, you should still take the time to read each option before moving on.

General Strategies

Tough Questions

If you are stumped on a problem or it appears too hard or too difficult, don't waste time. Move on! Remember though, if you can quickly check for obviously incorrect answer choices, your chances of guessing correctly are greatly improved. Before you completely give up, at least try to knock out a couple of possible answers. Eliminate what you can and then guess at the remaining answer choices before moving on.

Check Your Work

Since you will probably not know every term listed and the answer to every question, it is important that you get credit for the ones that you do know. Don't miss any questions through careless mistakes. If at all possible, try to take a second to look back over your answer selection and make sure you've selected the correct answer choice and haven't made a costly careless mistake (such as marking an answer choice that you didn't mean to mark). This quick double check should more than pay for itself in caught mistakes for the time it costs.

Pace Yourself

It's easy to be overwhelmed when you're looking at a page full of questions; your mind is confused and full of random thoughts, and the clock is ticking down faster than you would like. Calm down and maintain the pace that you have set for yourself. Especially as you get down to the last few minutes of the test, don't let the small numbers on the clock make you panic. As long as you are on track by monitoring your pace, you are guaranteed to have time for each question.

Don't Rush

It is very easy to make errors when you are in a hurry. Maintaining a fast pace in answering questions is pointless if it makes you miss questions that you would have gotten right otherwise. Test writers like to include distracting information and wrong answers that seem right. Taking a little extra time to avoid careless mistakes can make all the difference in your test score. Find a pace that allows you to be confident in the answers that you select.

KEEP MOVING

Panicking will not help you pass the test, so do your best to stay calm and keep moving. Taking deep breaths and going through the answer elimination steps you practiced can help to break through a stress barrier and keep your pace.

Final Notes

The combination of a solid foundation of content knowledge and the confidence that comes from practicing your plan for applying that knowledge is the key to maximizing your performance on test day. As your foundation of content knowledge is built up and strengthened, you'll find that the strategies included in this chapter become more and more effective in helping you quickly sift through the distractions and traps of the test to isolate the correct answer.

Now it's time to move on to the test content chapters of this book, but be sure to keep your goal in mind. As you read, think about how you will be able to apply this information on the test. If you've already seen sample questions for the test and you have an idea of the question format and style, try to come up with questions of your own that you can answer based on what you're reading. This will give you valuable practice applying your knowledge in the same ways you can expect to on test day.

Good luck and good studying!

Assessment

Anatomical Position

In any description of the human body, it is assumed to be in anatomical position. All of the terms used to describe the body do so relative to the anatomical position, which is the adopted standard in medicine. In this position, the body is standing with the feet facing forward. The feet are together, or slightly apart. The arms are to the sides, but not touching the sides. The palms are facing forward, so that the little finger is closest to the body. The thumbs point outward. It is important to remember that in the anatomical position, the thumb is lateral, and not medial. The head and eyes are facing forward.

Planes

The human body and its parts are often described in planes:

- A sagittal plane refers to a vertical plane parallel to the median which divides the body, or any body part, into right and left sections.
- A coronal plane is a vertical plane at right angles to the median which divides the body, or any body part, into anterior and posterior sections.
- A transverse plane is a horizontal plane which divides the body, or any body part, into upper and lower sections.
- A median plane is a sagittal plane which divides the body, or any body part, through the median into right and left halves.
- A frontal plane is another name for a coronal plane.

Bone Cells

The 3 major types of bones cells are osteocytes, osteoblasts, and osteoclasts. These cells act in concert to produce and destroy bone tissue, and keep the bones of the body healthy. Osteocytes are mature bone cells which develop from osteoblasts. They are the final stage in bone cell maturation, and the end of the bone cell lineage. They are non-dividing. Osteocytes are present in trabecular (cancellous) bone, and cortical bone. An osteoblast is a cell that manufactures bone. The osteoblast accomplishes this by producing a matrix which then mineralizes. They form all types of bone. An osteoclast is a bone cell which breaks down the bone matrix. It re-sorbs mineralized bone.

Bone Anatomy

Bone tissue is a type of connective tissue. The 2 types of bone tissue are compact (cortical) bone, and cancellous (spongy or trabecular) bone. Compact bone surrounds the marrow cavity, and is hard and dense. The ends of bones are composed of cancellous bone, which also lines the medullary cavity found in long bones. Cancellous bone appears spongy. Bone is surrounded by the periosteum. The periosteum is divided into 2 layers. New blood cells are produced in the inner layer of the periosteum. Nerves and blood vessels within the periosteum provide nourishment for the underlying bone, but are not sufficient to provide all the nourishment needed by the bone cortex. The periosteum also helps protect the bone from infection. The spaces in cancellous bone contain bone marrow. The medullary cavity is lined with a tissue called the endosteum. The medullary cavity contains a blood supply for the bone.

Bone Types

The skeleton is composed of long bones, short bones, flat bones, irregular bones, and sesamoid (round) bones. Examples of long bones are the humerus, and the femur. The shaft of a long bone, which is called the diaphysis, is made up of compact bone. The ends of a long bone are called the epiphyses, and these are made up of cancellous bone. The epiphyses are the sites of bone growth. Short bones are found in groups, and aid in movement. This type of bone is found in the wrist and ankle. Examples of flat bones are the ribs, scapula, sternum, and cranial bones. The vertebrae, facial bones, and skull bones are irregular bones. Sesamoid bones are located within a tendon. The patella, for example, is a sesamoid bone.

Facial Bones

There are 14 facial bones. They are responsible for face shape, and have sites of attachment for the jaw muscles, and the muscles of facial expression. The facial bones include the following: 1) 2 maxillae; 2) 2 palatine bones; 3) 2 zygomatic bones; 4) 2 lacrimal bones; 5) 2 nasal bones; 5) the mandible; and 6) 2 inferior nasal conchae. The maxillae form the upper jaw and hold the upper teeth. The palatine bones are found behind the maxillae and form part of the nasal cavity, and part of the hard palate. The zygomatic bones are the cheek bones. The lacrimal bones are located in the inner corner of the eye orbit. The nasal bones are seen as the bridge of the nose. The vomer is located in the nasal cavity and forms the nasal septum. The mandible is the lower jaw. The nasal conchae are in the nasal cavity.

Cranium Bones

The cranium encloses and protects the brain. The cranium has attachment points for the muscles that allow chewing, and the muscles that allow movement of the head. There are eight bones in the cranium. These are as follows: 1) the frontal bone; 2) 2 parietal bones, 3) the occipital bone; 4) 2 temporal bones; 5) the sphenoid bone; and 5) the ethmoid bone. These bones are attached by immovable joints called sutures. The frontal bone is located on the anterior part of the cranium. The 2 parietal bones make up the top and sides of the cranium. The occipital bone is found at the base of the cranium. The 2 temporal bones are found at the sides of the cranium. The sphenoid bone forms part of the base and sides of the cranium. The ethmoid bone is divided into 2 parts, with one on each side of the nasal cavity.

Vertebra

The vertebrae have different shapes, but they all have characteristics in common. The anterior part of the vertebra is thick and round, and is called the body. These vertebral bodies are separated by the intervertebral disks. Two projections called peduncles extend posteriorly from each vertebra. Attached to each peduncle is a lamina. These 2 laminae fuse in back to form the spinous process. The peduncles, laminae, and spinous process form the vertebral arch. The spinal cord passes through this arch. The transverse process is located between the peduncles and laminae, and projects laterally and inferiorly. The transverse process is a point of attachment for ligaments and muscles. The superior and inferior articulating processes extend from each vertebral arch. The latter two processes serve as attachments for the ligaments that connect adjacent vertebrae.

Vertebral Column

The vertebral column extends from the skull to the pelvis. It is comprised of bony vertebrae separated by intervertebral disks of cartilage. The vertebrae are tied together by ligaments. The vertebral column protects the spinal cord which travels through it via the vertebral foramen. There are 33 vertebrae in the spinal column, and they are divided into regions of differing numbers. The vertebrae are referred to by their location in the column. For example, the first cervical vertebra (the atlas) is referred to as C1, and the second cervical vertebra (the axis) is referred to as C2. From superior to inferior, these are as follows: cervical; thoracic, lumbar, sacral, and coccygeal. There are 7 cervical vertebrae, 12 thoracic vertebrae, and 5 lumbar vertebrae. The sacrum consists of 5 bones which fuse when adulthood is reached. The coccyx is composed of 4 fused vertebrae.

Pectoral Girdle Bones

The bones making up the pectoral girdle are the clavicle (collarbone) and scapula. There is one each of these bones on each side of the body. The clavicle is a long thin bone with 2 curves. It keeps the shoulder in place. One end of the bone attaches laterally to the acromion process of the scapula. The other end of the bone attaches medially to the manubrium of the sternum. The clavicle is easily broken. The scapula is commonly called the shoulder blade. It is a broad, triangular shaped flat bone. A scapula has three surfaces called fossae which serve as attachment points for muscle. The important sites on the scapula are the acromion process, the coracoid process, and the glenoid fossa. The coracoid process is an attachment point for the biceps. The humerus attaches to the glenoid fossa.

Thorax Bones

The bones in the thorax include the ribs, and the sternum. These structures protect the visceral organs, and aid in breathing. The human body contains 12 ribs attached to the 12 thoracic vertebrae. These bones are curved and slightly flattened. The first 7 ribs are called true ribs, as they are connected directly to the sternum by the costal cartilage. The next three ribs are referred to as the false ribs because they are not connected directly to the sternum. The cartilages of these ribs join together, and attach to the seventh costal cartilage. The last 2 ribs are not attached to the sternum, and are called floating ribs. The sternum is the breastbone. It is flat and divided into 3 parts: the upper manubrium, the middle body, and the xiphoid process. The sternal notch can be felt at the top of the sternum at the bottom of the throat.

Lower Arm Bones

The bones in the lower arm are the radius and ulna. The radius is the larger of the 2 bones in the lower arm, and it extends from the elbow to the wrist. It lies on the same side of the limb as the thumb. The proximal end of the radius is disk shaped, and articulates with the capitulum of the humerus. It also attaches at the proximal end to the radial notch of the ulna. The arrangement permits the radius to rotate around the ulna. The distal end of the radius articulates with the wrist via the articular facets. The ulna is attached to the humerus at the trochlear notch. On the distal end, the ulna articulates with the radius at the ulnar notch. The ulna connects to the wrist at the styloid process. The radius and ulna are connected by the interosseous membrane.

Upper Arm Bones

The bone of the upper arm is called the humerus. It is the largest bone in the arm, extending from the scapula to the elbow. The proximal end, which is called the head of the humerus, fits into the glenoid fossa. Two processes, called the greater and lesser tuberosities, are located below the head of the humerus. An area just below the tubercles, called the surgical neck, is a common site for fractures. The distal end of the humerus has 2 condyles. The lateral of these condyles is called the capitulum and it articulates with the head of the radius. The medical condyle is called the trochlea, and it articulates with the ulna. Above the condyles, the humerus flares out forming 2 epicondyles. The medial epicondyle is commonly called the funny bone, as the ulnar nerve is located at this site.

Phalangeal Bones

There are 14 phalangeal bones forming the fingers and thumbs. The phalanges articulate with the metacarpals. There are 3 bones in each finger (proximal, middle, and distal), and 2 bones in the thumb (proximal, and distal). Each bone is called a phalanx. Starting from the thumb, the phalanges are named according to their relative position to the metacarpals. The phalanx in the thumb closest to the metacarpal is phalanx I proximal. The other phalanx of the thumb is phalanx I distal. The phalanges of the little finger are called phalanx V proximal, phalanx V middle, and phalanx V distal. Like the metacarpals, the phalanges are long bones, and are cylindrical.

Carpals and Metacarpals

There are 8 carpal bones in the wrist arranged in 2 rows of 4. In the distal row, the bones are arranged in the following order from the lateral side to the medial side: trapezium, trapezoid, capitate, and hamate. A small bony projection on the distal end of the hamate is used in the identification of this bone. The projection is called the hamulus. The proximal row of bones contains the scaphoid (navicular), lunate, triquetrum, and pisiform. All of the carpal bones are short bones, except the pisiform, which is a sesamoid bone. The most commonly fractured carpal bone is the scaphoid. There are 5 metacarpal bones in the palm. Roman numerals are used to identify the five metacarpals. The metacarpals are long bones and are cylindrical. They number from 1 – V beginning with the thumb.

Hip, Femur, and Patella

The ball-and-socket joint of the hip is formed by the articulation of the acetabulum of the innominate bone, and the head of the femur. The acetabulum is found at the junction of the ilium, ischium, and pubis. The femur is the largest bone in the human body, and reaches from the hip to the knee. The greater and lesser trochanters, and the femoral head and neck make up the proximal end of the femur. The distal part of the femur ends in the lateral and medial condyles. These 2 condyles articulate with the condyles of the proximal end of the tibia and form the knee joint. The lateral and medial condyles are separated by a depression, called the patellar surface or groove, which provides an articular surface for the patella. The patella is a triangular shaped sesamoid bone which protects and strengthens the knee.

Pelvic Bones

The midline of pelvic girdle is formed by the sacrum and the coccyx. On either side of this midline complex is an os coxae. The os coxae is also referred to as the innominate bone. The os coxae is the result of the fusion of 3 bones, which are separate in children. These bones are the ilium, ischium, and pubis. The ilium is the largest of these bones, and forms the superior part of the pelvis. The ilium has a ridge which is called the iliac crest. Bone is often harvested from this area for bone grafts. The ischium makes up the inferior part of the pelvic girdle. The pubis is the anterior part of the pelvic girdle. The pubic bones are joined at the midline by a disk of cartilage to form the pubic symphysis. Women have wider and shallower pelvic girdles than do men.

Ankle and Foot Bones

There are 7 tarsal bones which are arranged in 2 rows. From lateral to medial, the bones in the proximal row are the calcaneous, talus and navicular. In the distal row, there are 4 bones. From lateral to medial these are the cuboid, medial cuneiform, intermediate cuneiform, and lateral cuneiform. These bones vary widely in shape and size. The largest of these bones is the calcaneous, or heel bone. The 5 metatarsals are the equivalent of the metacarpals. The metatarsals are numbered with Roman numerals beginning with the big toe. Metatarsals I, II, and, III articulate with the medial, intermediate, and lateral cuneiforms respectively. Metatarsals IV and V articulate with the cuboid. There are 14 phalanges in the feet. The big toe, known as the hallux, consists of 2 phalanges. The other toes have 3 phalanges each. They are numbered as the fingers, beginning with the big toe.

Tibia and Fibula

The tibia and fibula are long bones. The tibia, commonly called the shinbone, is the larger of the 2 bones in the lower leg. The tibia is the weight bearing bone and is located on the medial side. On the proximal end of the tibia are the medial and lateral condyles which articulate with the condyles of the femur and form the knee joint. The knee joint is cushioned by the crescent shaped lateral and medial menisci located on the tibia. The medial malleolus, on the distal part of the tibia, articulates with the talus bone contributing to the ankle joint. The fibula is a thin nonweight-bearing bone. It serves to stabilize the ankle joint. The lateral malleolus, on the distal end of the bone, articulates with the talus bone, forming part of the ankle joint.

Joint Types

Joints are classified according the way in which they move. The three types of joints are as follows: 1) immovable; 2) slightly movable; and 3) freely movable. An immovable joint is called a synarthrosis. The bones in this type of joint are in close contact, and separated by a thin cartilage. The cranial bones are separated by immovable joints. A slightly movable joint is called an amphiarthrosis. The pubic symphysis and the vertebral joints are examples of slightly movable joints. A freely movable joint is called a diarthrosis. This type of joint is also called a synovial joint. There are 6 types of freely movable joints. There are as follows: 1) ball-and-socket joints; 2) condyloid joints; 3) gliding joints; 4) hinge joints; 5) pivot joints; and 6) saddle joints.

Ball-and-Socket and Condyloid Joints

The ball-and-socket joint permits the widest range of motion of all the joint types. A ball-shaped head on one bone fits into a cup-shaped socket of another bone. This joint permits movement in all directions, and rotation. The hip and shoulder are ball-and-socket joints. A condyloid joint permits movement on one plane and some lateral movement. The condyle of 1 bone fits into the fossa of another bone. An example is the temperomandibular joint. A gliding joint permits twisting, and motion side-to-side. The bones in a gliding joint are either flat, or slightly curved. The carpals of the wrist form a gliding joint. A hinge joint allows movement in one direction. The concave surface of 1 bone articulates with the concave surface of another bone. The elbow is a hinge joint. A pivot joint permits rotational only. A saddle joint allows movement on a number of planes.

Soft Tissues of the Shoulder Joint

The rotator cuff consists of 4 muscles that stabilize the shoulder joint and permit motion of various kinds. These muscles are the infraspinatus, the subscapularis, the supraspinatus, and the teres minor. The origin of these muscles is the scapula. These muscles insert on the tubercles of the humerus. The tendons of the supraspinatus, infraspinatus, and teres minor muscles insert on the greater tubercle of the humerus. The tendon of the subscapular muscle inserts on the lesser tubercle. The acromion of the scapula is the site of origin for the deltoid. The deltoid inserts on the deltoid tuberosity of the humeral shaft. Tears to the muscles of the rotator cuff, dislocation, and ligament damage are common shoulder injuries. The bursae of the shoulder are found between the muscles of the rotator cuff and the outer shoulder muscles. The shoulder is a ball-and-socket joint capable of internal rotation, abduction, and adduction.

Soft Tissue Structures of the Elbow

The humerus, radius, and ulna form this hinge joint. The elbow is a very stable joint. The joint is supported by the ulnar collateral ligament, the radial collateral ligament, the anterior ligament, and the posterior ligament. The annular ligament keeps the radius in contact with the ulna at the radial notch. The muscle in front of the joint is the Brachialis. The muscles behind the joint are the Triceps brachii, and the Anconaeus. The muscles laterally are the Supinator, and the common tendon of origin of the Extensor muscles. The medial muscles are the Flexor carpi ulnaris, and the common tendon of origin of the Flexor muscles. Simply, the biceps flexes the joint, and the triceps extends the joint. The elbow joint can flex, extend, pronate, and supinate. The articular surfaces of the elbow joint share a synovial membrane which encloses the joint.

Soft Tissue Structures of the Hip

The hip is a ball-and-socket joint, and is the most mobile of the joints in the lower extremity. The joint is formed by the articulation of the acetabulum of the pelvis with the head of the femur. The acetabulum is surrounded by a fibrocartilaginous cuff which makes the cup of the acetabulum deeper. This makes it harder for the joint to dislocate. The hip joint is tied together by 3 ligaments. These are as follows: the iliofemoral ligament (ligament of Bigelow), pubofemoral ligament, and the ischiofemoral ligament. The iliofemoral ligament joins the pelvis and femur. This ligament prevents the joint from extending excessively. The pubofemoral ligament passes from the pubis to the femur. The ischiofemoral ligament stretches from the acetabular rim to the femur. The muscles of the hips allow extension, medial and lateral rotation, adduction, flexion, and abduction. The hip is enclosed by an extensive fibrous capsule.

Soft Tissue Structures of the Knee

The patella is located within the quadriceps tendon, which stretches from the quadriceps muscles, and connects to the superior portion of the patella. The patella ligament (sometimes referred to as the patellar tendon) originates on the inferior part of the patella and inserts below onto the tuberosity of the tibia. Together, the quadriceps tendon and the patella tendon stabilize the patella and straighten the knee. The anterior and posterior cruciate ligaments also help stabilize the knee joint. They are located in the middle of the joint in the intercondylar area. The posterior cruciate ligament, known as the PCL, prevents the anterior displacement of the femur relative to the tibia. It attaches to the medial condyle of the femur, and the posterior surface of the tibia at the midline. The anterior cruciate ligament, known as the ACL, prevents the posterior displacement of the femur relative to the tibia. It prevents the knee from hyperextending, and limits the extent that the femur can rotate medially when the foot is planted. It attaches to the posterior lateral condyle of the femur, and to a notch between the tibial condyles. The tibia is topped by menisci.

Menisci of the Knee

Each knee has 2 menisci. The lateral and medical menisci act as shock absorbers for the knee. These structures are fluid-filled crescent-shaped disks of cartilage which sit on the upper surface of the tibia. The borders of the menisci are attached to the lining of the knee. Clinically, the meniscus is divided into three sections. These are the anterior horn, body, and the posterior horn. Except at its borders, the menisci are avascular, meaning they have no blood supply. Because of this, small tears at the edge of the menisci may heal, but the inner part of the menisci cannot repair itself if damaged. Meniscal tears usually occur as a result of twisting injuries, or a direct hit to the side of the knee. The menisci dry out with normal aging, and tears may result. The medial meniscus tears more often than the lateral meniscus.

The medial meniscus is almost semi-circular in shape. The anterior end of the medial meniscus, which is thin and pointed, is attached to the anterior intercondyloid fossa of the tibia. The posterior end of the meniscus is attached to the posterior intercondyloid fossa of the tibia. Due to its attachments, the medial meniscus cannot slide around very much, and tears under stress.

The lateral meniscus is almost circular, and covers more of the articular surface of the tibia than does the medial meniscus. The lateral side of the meniscus has a groove to accommodate the tendon of the Popliteus. The anterior portion attaches in front of the tibia's intercondyloid eminence. The posterior end attaches behind the tibia's intercondyloid eminence, and in front of the posterior part of the medial meniscus. One part of the lateral meniscus is not attached. Under stress, it is more likely to move than tear.

Knee Capsule

The capsule of the knee is attached to the femur, tibia, and fibula at several locations. Proximally, it is attached to the femur at the lateral and medial condyles. Distally, it is attached to the tibia at the lateral and medial condyles. It is also attached to the superior part of the fibula. The capsule is stabilized by the patellar and quadriceps tendons, the medial and lateral collateral ligaments, and the popliteus and gastrocnemius muscles. The capsule has several thickened areas which form internal ligaments. These internal ligaments are the short internal ligament, the arcuate popliteal ligament (short external ligament), and the medial and lateral patellar retinacular fibers. The medial patellar reticular fibers prevent the patella from dislocating laterally. Anatomically, there is a deficiency of the capsule at the back of the knee. Due to this, the synovium may herniate under pressure, and form a Baker's cyst.

Carpal Tunnel

The carpal tunnel is a narrow passageway in the wrist formed by the carpal bones, and the transverse carpal ligament on the inside of the wrist. The circumference of the tunnel is about the same as that of the thumb. The median nerve and 9 flexor tendons of the hand travel through this tunnel. The carpal tunnel protects these structures. The size of the tunnel can be decreased significantly through flexion of the wrist. Carpal tunnel syndrome is caused by the compression of the median nerve in the tunnel. This compression may result from the swelling, or thickening of the transverse carpal ligament. An acquired or congenital deformity can also cause such a compression.

Soft Tissues of the Wrist

The wrist joint is formed by the distal end of the radius, and the proximal carpals bones. This is the radiocarpal joint. The midcarpal joint, which is found between the proximal and distal row of carpal bones, is closely associated.

The ligaments associated with the wrist include the volar radiocarpal ligament, the dorsal radiocarpal ligament, the ulnar collateral ligament, and the radial collateral ligament. The synovial membrane of the joint extends from the distal end of the radius to the proximal ends of the articular surfaces of the carpal bones. This synovial membrane has numerous folds in it, and is loose to allow movement. The wrist joint can adduct, abduct, extend, flex and circumduct. Wrist extension occurs mainly at the midcarpal joint, while wrist flexion occurs mainly at the radiocarpal joint. The wrist and hand are capable of extremely fine movement due to the number of muscles.

Ankle Joint

The true ankle joint contain 3 bones. These are the tibia, the fibula, and the talus. The true ankle joint allows dorsiflexion and plantarflexion. Underneath the true ankle joint is the subtalar joint which is composed of the talus and calcaneous. The subtalar joint permits side-to-side motion. On the lateral side, the tibiofibular ligament attaches to the tibia and fibula. The lateral collateral ligaments connect the fibula and the calcaneous; these ligaments provide lateral stability. On the medial side of the ankle the deltoid ligaments join the tibia to the talus and to the calcaneous. These ligaments stabilize the ankle medially. Excessive movement of the subtalar joint often leads to injuries to these ligaments. The best known of the tendons moving the ankle is the Achilles tendon which runs down the back of the ankle, connecting the muscles in the calf to the heel. This tendon is often injured.

Normal Bone Healing

A fractured bone should normally heal within 8 – 12 weeks. To ensure good healing, the fracture should be properly aligned, and immobilized by internal, or external fixation. There are 5 stages to normal bone healing. These are as follows: 1) inflammation, 2) cellular proliferation, 3) callus formation, 4) ossification, and 5) remodeling. The inflammatory stage of healing lasts about 2 days. A blood clot, called the fracture hematoma is formed. The cellular proliferation stage begins on the second day post-injury. Macrophages debride the injured area. A fibrin mesh is produced which seals the edges of the fractured bones. The fibrin mesh allows capillary and fibroblastic ingrowth. Fibroblasts and osteoblasts form a periosteal callus. The callus formation stage continues for 3 - 4 weeks. During this stage, the bone fragments grow together. The ossification stage lasts 3 - 4 months. The new tissue calcifies. The remodeling stage is normal bone maintenance.

Pathological Bone Healing

Bone healing can be disrupted at any stage. Inadequate immobilization of the injury, distraction of the bone fragments, inadequate blood supply, infection, and interposition of soft tissues can all interfere with proper healing. If the bone is poorly immobilized, the formation of the hematoma can be disturbed. Distracted fragments of bone are separated and do not come into contact. Granular tissue may fill the space between the bone fragments, and interfere with healing. Also distraction may decrease the blood supply to the site of injury. In a case of distraction, soft tissue may fill the gap, and cover the ends of the fracture interfering with hematoma and callus formation. Vascular necrosis of the bone may occur when the blood supply is not reestablished. Advancing age, poor nutrition, and hormone imbalances can affect healing adversely.

Fibrosis, Erysipelas, Cornification, Keratosis, and Edema

These conditions can occur with lymphedema. Fibrosis is the hardening of soft tissue. Erysipelas, which means red skin in Greek, is the result of an acute streptococcal infection of the skin. The infection causes inflammation, and involves the fat underlying the affected skin. Cornification involves the change of normal skin cells into a hard material such as keratin. Keratosis involves the growth of thick scaly bumps on the skin. Edema is the accumulation of interstitial fluid in any soft tissue resulting in a swollen appearance. It results from the increased secretion of interstitial fluid, or a problem in removing it from the tissue. Edema used to be called dropsy, or hydropsy.

Laboratory Tests

The erythrocyte sedimentation test measures how long it takes red blood cells to settle, or fall, to the bottom of a test tube. During a time of inflammation red blood cells have an elevated rate of sedimentation, meaning they settle faster. This test is used in the diagnosis of inflammatory conditions, such as rheumatoid arthritis, and ankylosing spondylitis. The human leukocyte antigens are proteins occurring on white blood cells. The presence of HLA-B27 is indicative of ankylosing spondylitis. The latex fixation test detects rheumatoid factors, and so is used in diagnosing rheumatoid arthritis. Rheumatoid factors test measures the amount rheumatoid factor in the blood. Presence of this is indicative of rheumatoid arthritis.

An analysis of synovial fluid is used to differentiate between osteoarthritis, rheumatoid arthritis, or gout. These disorders have similar symptoms, but rheumatoid factors are present in synovial fluid only in a case of rheumatoid arthritis.

The antinuclear antibody test is used to diagnose autoimmune disorders. Antinuclear antibodies are produced in reaction to the body's own nuclear material. These antibodies are present in a case of autoimmune disease, such as systemic lupus erythematosus.

Bence Jones protein is produced in a case of multiple myeloma. This protein is produced by malignant plasma cells, and can be detected in the urine.

Cultures are used to identify disease causing microorganisms. Infectious diseases can be diagnosed using cultures.

Although alkaline phosphatase is necessary for building new bone, increased levels of alkaline phosphatase in the blood indicates bone disease. Possible diseases indicated by a raised alkaline phosphatase level include multiple myeloma, osteomalacia, and osteogenic sarcoma.

Calcium and phosphorus are components of normal bone, but elevated levels in the blood and urine indicate disease. Diseases diagnosed by elevated levels of calcium and phosphorus include osteoporosis, and osteomalacia.

An abnormally high level of serum urate is suggestive of gout, but high levels of urate may also be indicative of other diseases such as lymphoma, leukemia, and hemolytic anemia. A normal serum urate level does not necessarily rule out gout.

Elevated levels of urinary uric acid may indicate gout.

Fractures

The following are various types of fracture:

- A comminuted fracture is one in which the bone is broken into more than 2 pieces.
- A depressed fracture occurs when the bone is pushed in. It is often seen in skull fractures.
- A displaced fracture refers to a fracture in which the bones are out of alignment.
- An intra-articular fracture refers to an injury in which the bones inside a joint are fractured.
- A simple fracture refers to a situation in which the bone is in normal anatomical alignment, is not piercing the skin.
- A spontaneous fracture is refers to a break that occurred without trauma. It is also called a pathological fracture.
- A stellate fracture is one in which additional fractures radiate from a central fracture.
- A spiral fracture is also called a torsion fracture. This type of fracture is caused by the twisting of the bone. A spiral fracture is a fracture of a long bone that extends up and down the bone like a corkscrew. This type of fracture is highly unstable. It is often misdiagnosed as an oblique fracture.
- A greenstick fracture involves a break on only one side of the bone cortex. This is an incomplete fracture that is most often seen in children who have softer, more malleable bones. Greenstick fractures occur from the bending of the bone. These fractures are extremely stable, and heal well.
- An impacted fracture is one in which one end of the broken bone is driven into the other broken end. This type of fracture is difficult to see in an x-ray because the transradiant line usually seen with a fracture is missing.
- An agenetic fracture is a spontaneous fracture that results from less than ideal osteogenesis.
- An atrophic fracture is a spontaneous fracture that results from bone atrophy.
- A buttonhole fracture is a fracture in which the bone is penetrated by a projectile, causing a hole in the bone. It is also called a perforating fracture.
- A capillary fracture is one that appears as a thin line in a radiograph, as the bone fragments are not separated.
- A chisel fracture is one where a slanted piece of bone is detached from the head of the radius.
- A direct is one that occurs at the site of an injury.
- A dyscrasic fracture is one that occurs due to the weakening of the bone from disease.
- A closed fracture is one that is not associated with an open wound.
- A complete fracture is one which goes through the entire cross section of the bone.

- A compound fracture is one in which the broken end of the bone penetrates the skin, exposing the bone.
- A dislocation fracture occurs near a joint and involves a co-occurring dislocation of the joint.
- A fissure fracture is a crack in the surface of a bone that does not extend through the bone.
- An incomplete fracture is one that does not extend through the entire bone.
- An insufficiency fracture is a stress fracture that occurs when bone that is abnormally thin is placed under stress.
- A sprain fracture refers to a situation in which a piece of bone is pulled away when a tendon is separated from its insertion point.
- A trophic fracture results from nutritional deficits.
- A lead pipe fracture involves the compression of the cortex on one side of the bone, and a crack on the opposite side of the bone.
- A neoplastic fracture is one that occurs in a bone weakened by a malignancy.
- A neurogenic fracture is one that occurs in a bone weakened by a neurological disorder.
- A nightstick fracture is a fracture of the shaft of the ulna. It obtained this name because it occurs during the blocking of a downward blow of an object such as a nightstick.
- A periarticular fracture is one that occurs near a joint.
- A pressure fracture is one that occurs due to pressure placed on the bone by a tumor.
- A resecting fracture is one in which a fragment of bone is removed by a violent action.
- An intraperiosteal does not involve a break in the periosteum.
- An endocrine fracture is a fracture that occurs as a result of the bone weakening from an endocrine disorder.
- A fissure fracture is one that involves the surface of the bone, but does not go all the way through it.
- A grenade-thrower's fracture is a fracture of the humerus caused by the muscular actions involved in throwing a heavy object (such as a grenade).
- An indirect fracture is one that is at some distance from the location of an injury.
- An inflammatory fracture is one that results when a bone is weakened by inflammation.
- An intracapsular fracture is one that occurs within the joint capsule.
- A segmental fracture is a double fracture.
- A splintered fracture is a comminuted fracture where the bones are broken into sharp thin pieces.
- A subcapital fracture is the fracture of a bone underneath its head.
- A subcutaneous fracture is one that does not penetrate the skin.
- A subperiosteal fracture is one in which the break does not penetrate the periosteum, and the shape and alignment of the bone are not changed.
- A supracondylar fracture is one involving the lower end of the shaft of the humerus.
- A transcondylar fracture is a fracture involving the condyles of the humerus in which the fracture line crosses the fossae. The fracture extends into the joint capsule.
- A willow fracture is a greenstick fracture.
- A basal fracture is one involving the neck of the femur near the trochanters.
- A bumper fracture is a fracture that involves one or both of the lower extremities below the knee. It is called a bumper fracture as it is sometimes caused by an automobile bumper.
- Duverney's fracture is a fracture of the ilium.
- A paratrooper's fracture is a fracture of the posterior part of the tibial articular margin, and/or of the malleoli.
- A petrochanteric fracture is a fracture of the greater trochanter of the femur.
- A Segond fracture is one involving the iliotibial band.

- A Shepherd's fracture is a fracture of the external tubercle of the talus (astragalus).
- A Stieda's fracture is a fracture of the femur at the internal condyle.
- A sprinter's fracture is an avulsion fracture of the anterior superior, or inferior, spine of the ilium. In this injury, a piece of bone is pulled off by muscular effort.
- Wagstaffe's fracture is a fracture with an accompanying dislocation of the medial malleolus.

Transverse and Oblique Fractures

A transverse fracture is a straight break that runs across the long axis of the bone at a right angle. These are often referred to as simple fractures. Transverse fractures often result from a direct blow to the bone. This type of fracture tends to stay in alignment. An oblique fracture is one in which the fracture line is at an angle to the long axis of the bone. These fractures are of note because they are less stable than transverse fractures, and as such, are more likely to displace. They are also rare. Spiral fractures are often misdiagnosed as oblique fractures. An oblique fracture is caused by a twisting motion.

Stress, Butterfly, and Avulsion Fractures

A stress fracture is a crack in the bone which often does not show up when first examined with an x-ray. It is also called a March fracture. This kind of fracture results from too much stress being placed on the bone.

A butterfly fracture is a type of comminuted fracture in which the bone is broken into fragments. A butterfly fracture involves 2 fragments on each side of a central fragment. The fractured pieces resemble a butterfly. The type of fracture is usually caused by a high energy force. An avulsion fracture occurs at the point where a tendon or ligament attaches to a bone. The tendon or ligament pulls away from the bone, and in the process breaks off a piece of bone. The usual cause is direct force from having the extremity bend abnormally.

Bennett's Fracture

Bennett's fracture is a type of intra-articular fracture which involves a dislocation. It is an oblique fracture of the base of metacarpal of the thumb. To be considered a Bennett's fracture, the fracture must extend into the carpometacarpal (CMC) joint. Distraction of the fractured bone ends occurs due muscular action. The abductor pollicis longus muscle shifts the metacarpal shaft laterally. A portion of the metacarpal bone remains in articulation with the trapezium. Keeping the fragments in alignment for proper healing is a challenge. It may be possible to treat some of these injuries by closed reduction, and casting. External fixation with pins, or open reduction and internal fixation may be necessary. The injury occurs due to a forceful abduction of the thumb. It is often seen in football players. The injury may result in arthritis.

Barton's Fracture and Reverse Barton's Fracture

Barton's fracture is an intra-articular oblique fracture of the distal radius involving the radiocarpal joint. It is a comminuted fracture. Barton's fracture is associated with dislocation of the radiocarpal joint. The fracture line of a Barton's facture extends across the dorsal rim of the radius and runs into the wrist joint. A fracture of the radio styloid process often accompanies a Barton's fracture. This is an unstable fracture, and readily redisplaces. It often occurs as the result of a fall forward onto an extended hand. It is the most commonly occurring fracture/dislocation of the wrist joint. Nonoperative treatment of this fracture often fails. A Barton's fracture is often confused clinically with a Colles fracture. A reverse Barton's fracture is much like a Barton's fracture except that the fracture lies along the volar rim of the distal radius instead of the dorsal rim.

Rolando's Fracture

Like Bennett's fracture, Rolando's fracture is a fracture/dislocation of the first metacarpal (thumb) at the base of the bone. It is a comminuted, intra-articular fracture. Three fracture fragments are usually involved which form a T or Y pattern. A Rolando's fracture is differentiated from Bennett's by the fact that Bennett's fracture is not comminuted. If the bone is in many small fragments, non-surgical treatment by immobilization is often advised. If the bone is broken into large fragments the fracture is often treated with open reduction, and internal fixation. This type of fracture is difficult to treat. This is a relatively uncommon type of fracture. Like Bennett's fracture, Rolando's fracture is caused by a forceful abduction of the thumb. It often results in osteoarthritis.

Buckle Fracture

A buckle fracture, also called a torus fracture, is a type of incomplete fracture. The cortex of the bone is compressed causing a buckle on the compressed side. The other side of the bone is undamaged. There are two types of buckle fractures. These are the classic buckle fracture and the angled buckle fracture. These injuries are very similar. The classic buckle fracture involves the outward buckling of the cortex of the bone on one side. The angled buckle fracture involves the simple angling of the cortex. This type of fracture is stable, and heals well with casting. It is most often seen in children because their bones are softer. The injury may be caused by a fall on an outstretched arm.

Chauffeur's Fracture

A chauffeur's fracture, also called Hutchinson's fracture, is an intra-articular oblique fracture of the radial styloid process. The fracture occurs on the articular surface of the radius, and generally extends laterally from the meeting point of the lunate and scaphoid fossae. The radial styloid process may be pulled away from the radius by the ligaments. A dislocation of the lunate may occur with this fracture. The injury is called a chauffeur's fracture as it was often caused by the kickback from the starting crank of a car. This injury is much less common today, but still occurs during falls on the ball of the thumb, and during forceful ulnar deviation and forceful supination of the wrist. This fracture is treated by casting, or fixation with hardware.

Colles Fracture

A Colles fracture is also called a Colles' fracture. This is a fracture of the distal metaphysis of the radius in which the fracture fragment is displaced dorsally (upward). The articular surface of the radius may be involved. The ulna styloid may also be fractured. A forced dorsiflexion of the wrist may lead to this type of fracture; a Colles fracture results most often from a fall forward onto an extended hand. This type of fracture is particularly common in elderly individuals. If there is minimal displacement, the fracture can be treated by casting. If the displacement is more severe, an open reduction may be necessary. A Colles fracture may be indicative of osteoporosis. Colles fracture is associated with a higher risk of experiencing a hip fracture.

Boxer's Fracture

A boxer's fracture involves a fracture in the fifth metacarpal (little finger). The fracture occurs at the distal metaphysic. It is called a boxer's fracture as it may result from punching an object with a closed fist. The metacarpal may be fractured into fragments, or displaced. This type of fracture does not generally extend into the joint, so arthritis is not likely to result. The loss of the knuckle of the fifth metacarpal occurs with this type of fracture. In addition, the injury may lead to the malrotation of the fifth metacarpal. This is evident when a fist is made, and the fifth metacarpal overlaps the ring finger. This weakens the grip of the hand. The degree of angulation of the fracture determines treatment. Casting with, or without external fixation may be used if the degree of angulation is small, but these fractures often require open reduction, and internal fixation.

MALLET FRACTURE

Mallet fracture is a type of mallet finger. Mallet finger is a disruption, in any of the digits, of the extensor mechanism of the distal interphalangeal joint. The tendon and bone are both involved in extension, and disruption of either of these can lead to mallet finger. If the bone is involved, it is called a mallet fracture. The section of the bone involved is the dorsal base of the phalanx. This is an avulsion fracture, where a piece of bone is pulled away. This injury causes the finger to drop. A mallet finger is often cause by a forceful hyperextension. This condition often leads to a stiff finger. The condition is treated both by open and closed reduction.

SMITH'S FRACTURE

Smith's fracture (Smith fracture) is also referred to as a reverse Colles fracture. It involves a transverse fracture of the distal radius at the metaphysic. This fracture involves a palmar (volar) displacement of the distal fragment of the fracture. The Colles fracture involves a dorsal displacement. Smith's fracture occurs as a result of falling forward onto flexed wrists, as opposed to a Colles fracture which occurs from falling forward on extended wrists. Smith's fractures occur less frequently than Colles fractures. A Smith's fracture does not involve the joint. This is an unstable fracture. The type of treatment depends upon the severity of the injury. A closed reduction may be sufficient for fractures with little angulation and displacement. Open reduction and internal fixation may be required to treat fractures with significant angulation.

MONTEGGIA FRACTURE

A Monteggia fracture is a fracture of the proximal ulna with an accompanying dislocation of the radial head within the elbow joint. There are two types of Monteggia fracture. These are the extension and flexion Monteggia fractures. The type depends upon the displacement of the bone fragment. This fracture type is the result of force transmitted through the hand and forearm with the elbow bent. The radius is pulled away from the joint by the interosseous ligament. It often occurs from a fall forward onto an outstretched hand while the elbow is slightly flexed. It is necessary to repair the fracture to prevent the elbow joint from continuing to dislocate. Casting the fracture is not sufficient to prevent this. The treatment is usually open reduction and internal fixation.

GALEAZZI'S FRACTURE

Galeazzi's fracture is also called a reverse Monteggia fracture. It is a fracture/dislocation. It involves a fracture of the shaft of the radius between the middle and distal thirds, and a dislocation of the inferior radioulnar joint. The distal fragment of the radius is generally displaced toward the ulnar. The dislocation is generally dorsal, but may be palmar. There may be an accompanying avulsion fracture of the ulnar styloid process. This fracture is usually caused by a direct blow to the dorsal side of the wrist, or by a fall forward onto an outstretched arm when the forearm is pronated. In adults, closed reduction may fail. An open reduction using plates and screws is often necessary.

Review Video: Hand and Forearm Conditions
Visit mometrix.com/academy and enter code: 394915

DE QUERVAIN'S, MOORE'S, SKILLERN'S, AND WILSON'S

De Quervain's fracture is also called simply Quervain's fracture. It is a fracture of the navicular bone in conjunction with a volar dislocation of the lunate bone. Moore's fracture is a fracture of the distal portion of the radius with an accompanying dislocation of the ulnar head, and entrapment of the styloid process under the annular ligaments. Skillern's fracture is a complete fracture through the bottom third of the radius with an accompanying greenstick fracture of the bottom third of the ulna. Wilson's fracture is a fracture at the site of the proximal interphalangeal joint. A fibrous strip called the volar plate is found at this site. It is a part of the capsule of the joint. Wilson's fracture is an avulsion fracture at this site. This injury is caused by hyperextension of the joint.

Tuft Fracture

A Tuft fracture is a distal phalanx fracture. In other words it involves the fingertip. There are degrees of severity. Most of these are comminuted fractures with accompanying damage to the nail bed. The fracture may be open, or closed. The amount of damage to the nail determines the treatment. If the nail plate is unaffected, it is left in place, and the hematoma is drained through it. If the fracture is of the open variety where the nail bed is damaged or destroyed the nail is removed, and the bed repaired. If the finger is splinted, it is splinted in an extended position. Comminuted fractures and those with soft tissue damage have poorer prognoses. This fracture usually results from blunt trauma to the fingertip, or a crushing injury.

Pilon Fracture

A pilon fracture is a comminuted fracture of the distal end of the tibia. The fracture is oblique and extends medially and laterally, and to the articular surface of the tibiotalar joint. The fracture may involve the metaphysis and joint. There may be significant soft tissue damage. This is an impact injury caused by axial loading. These fractures result when the talus is driven with force into the tibial plafond. In this type of fracture, the cortical bone is fragmented by the impact. In a high impact injury, the fibula may be involved. Treatment if difficult, and this type of fracture often results in posttraumatic arthritis. High impact fractures tend to have a poor prognosis no matter the treatment.

Pott's Fracture, a Gosselin's Fracture, and a Maisonneuve Fracture

A Pott's fracture is a fracture dislocation of the ankle. This fracture is also known as a Dupuytren fracture. It is a fracture of the fibula above the ankle joint, and also often involves a fracture of the medial malleolus. The internal lateral ligament is often ruptured as well. The foot is displaced laterally. Gosselin's fracture is a v-shaped fracture of the distal tibia which extends to the ankle joint. A Maisonneuve fracture is a spiral fracture of the proximal third of the fibula. It also includes a disruption of the distal tibiofibular syndesmosis. A fracture of the tibia and a tear of the deltoid ligament may be associated with a Maisonneuve fracture.

Triplane Fracture

A triplane fracture, also called the Marmor-Lynn fracture, involves fractures of the epiphysis, physis, and metaphysis of the distal tibia. The fractures are vertical, transverse, and coronal respectively. The growth plate of the tibia is affected. A triplane fracture is produced by a twisting motion. The injury occurs when eversion of the foot puts stress on the distal lateral growth plate of the tibia. This is a common fracture in adolescents, and occurs before the closing of the growth plate. The severity of the injury is difficult to detect on radiographs. It is a Salter-Harris IV fracture. A CT scan or MRI should be performed if a triplane fracture is suspected. Closed reduction may be possible, but with more severe fractures, an open reduction may be necessary.

Tillaux Fracture

A Tillaux fracture is an avulsion fracture of the anterior lateral margin of the distal end of the tibia. It is a twisting injury, and occurs when the anterior tibiofibular ligament pulls a part of the tibia away from the bone. It is caused when the foot is forcefully turned laterally, or when the leg is forcefully turned medially on a planted foot. This injury is common in adolescents, but is rarely seen in adults. In adults, the ligament involved usually breaks instead of causing an avulsion injury. In children and adolescents, the ligament is stronger than the growth plate. The ligament injury sometimes seen in adults is called a Tillaux lesion. Treatment of these fractures often involves internal fixation. This injury is often caused by skateboarding accidents, and sliding in baseball. This is a Salter-Harris II fracture.

Jones Fracture

A Jones fracture is a fracture of the base of the fifth metatarsal at the junction of the metaphysic and diaphysis. The fracture generally extends into the intermetatarsal facet between the fourth and fifth metatarsals. The fracture produces pain in the middle and outer part of the foot, and causes difficulty walking. This fracture is often mistaken for a sprain. Diagnosis is made based on x-ray results. An undisplaced Jones fracture can be treated successfully with a cast, or walking boot. If the fracture is more severe, a screw can be used to hold the bones in place. This fracture may heal poorly due to the poor blood supply to the area. Also, the tendons may full the fragments apart.

Trimalleolar Fracture

A trimalleolar fracture, also called a Henderson fracture or a Cotton fracture, involves fractures of the medial and lateral malleoli of the tibia, and the posterior process of the tibia. The posterior process is not actually a malleolus, and therefore the name trimalleolar fracture is misleading. The 3 parts of the tibia mentioned all articulate with the talus bone. This is a fracture caused by severe trauma. A trimalleolar fracture is unstable, and the treatment is open reduction, and internal fixation. It is considered an orthopedic emergency. An ankle with a healing trimalleolor fracture is not able to bear weight even with internal fixation. Healing normally takes 6 weeks. The fracture is likely to lead to osteoarthritis.

Burst, Jefferson's, and Ping-Pong Fractures

A burst fracture is a fracture in which the body of the vertebra is crushed all around. The injury is severe as the bone fragments are likely to damage the spinal cord resulting in paralysis, or a lesser injury to the nerves. This type of fracture is the result of forceful pressure on the vertebral column. A Jefferson fracture involves unilateral or bilateral fractures of the first cervical vertebra at the anterior and posterior arches. This is an axial loading (compression) injuries. It is an unstable fracture. A ping-pong fracture is a depression fracture of the skull. It is called a ping-pong fracture as is resembles the depression that can be made on a ping-pong ball. This type of fracture occurs when the bones of the skull are soft, and so it is seen in newborns and infants. The ping-pong fracture can occur during delivery. They may resolve spontaneously.

Salter-Harris Fractures Type I, and II

Salter-Harris fractures are fractures of the growth plate (physis). They occur before the growth plates are closed. There are 5 categories of Salter-Harris fracture based on the type of damage to the bony structures. In a type I fracture the epiphysis of the bone is completely separated from the metaphysis. The physis (growth plate) remains attached to the epiphysis. This type of fracture is requires no reduction usually, and is casted. The fracture usually heals normally with no disturbance to growth. A type II fracture involves the partial separation of the epiphysis and physis from the metaphysis. The metaphysis is cracked. A type II fracture usually has to be reduced, and must be immobilized. This is the most common type of Salter-Harris fracture, and may cause shortening of the bone.

Le Fort Fractures

A Le Fort fracture involves the facial bones. It consists of a transverse fracture at the base of the upper jaw (maxillae). There are 3 types of le Fort fracture of increasing degrees of severity. A Le Fort fracture I, involves a transverse (horizontal) segmented fracture through the alveolar process of the maxilla. The detached portion of bone usually holds the teeth. This fracture is also called Guérin's fracture. A Le Fort fracture II is a bilateral or unilateral fracture of the maxilla. A pyramid shaped section of the body of the maxilla is separated from the rest of the facial skeleton. It is also called a pyramidal fracture. A Le Fort fracture III, involves the complete separation of the maxilla, and one or more facial bones from the rest of the facial skeleton. It is also called a craniofacial disjunction, and transverse facial fracture. These are blunt force injuries.

Peterson Classification of Growth Plate Fractures

The Peterson classification is an extension of the Salter-Harris classification of growth plate fractures. It is a newer classification, and adds a type VI fracture category. In the type VI fracture category, a part of the epiphysis, physis, and metaphysis is removed from the site. This type of fracture usually occurs with accidents involving heavy machinery, or gunshots wounds. An open wound, or compound fracture is usually associated with type VI fractures. Type VI fractures always necessitate surgery, and follow-up reconstructive or corrective surgery is very often required at a later date. As the growth plate is so damaged by the injury, bone growth is almost adversely affected. Prognosis is poor.

Salter-Harris Fractures Type III, IV and V

A Salter-Harris fracture type III is rare, and occurs usually at the distal portion of the tibia. The fracture extends through the epiphysis, and separates a portion of the epiphysis and physis from the metaphysis. It affects the articular surface of the bone. Surgery is sometimes necessary. Prognosis is relatively good, but some disability may result. The Salter-Harris fracture type IV extends across the physis, into the metaphysis. Surgery is necessary to repair the surface of the joint, and to align the physis. If perfect alignment is not attained and maintained, prognosis and poor, and growth will be affected. The Salter-Harris type IV usually occurs at the distal end of the humerus. The Salter-Harris type V fracture is the result of the crushing of the bone, and compression of the physis. Prognosis is poor, and the growth of the bone is stunted.

Tibial Plateau Fracture

A tibial plateau fracture used to be called fender, or bumper, fractures as they can be caused by impact from a car. The injury is usually caused, however, from a twisting injury, or lateral forces on the bone. The Schatzker classification system is used to describe 6 patterns of fracture. Type 1 fractures involve a split in the lateral tibial plateau. A Type II fracture is a split fracture with an accompanying depression at the lateral articular surface. Type II fractures involve a depression of the lateral tibial plateau. Type IV fractures are found in the medial tibial plateau. These may be split fractures with or without an associated depression fracture. Type V fractures involve splits through the medial plateau, and the lateral plateau. The Type VI fracture is the most serious, and involves a dissociation of the tibial plateau, and diaphysis.

Soft tissue damage is often associated with tibial plateau fractures. Cruciate ligaments, collateral ligaments, peroneal nerve injury, and popliteal artery occlusion may result from these fractures. Skin injuries are often associated with tibial plateau fractures, and osteomyelitis may result. Symptoms of this fracture type include excess fluid in the knee, pain, and stiffness of the joint. Tibial plateau fractures are easily diagnosed by x-ray. Depending on the severity of the fracture reduction may be nonsurgical, or surgical. Whatever the treatment, the joint may be unstable after healing die to damage to the ligaments. Damage to the cartilage and articular discontinuities may also result from these fractures. Three is a high risk of osteoarthritis.

Inter-Trochanteric Fracture

An inter-trochanteric fracture occurs between the greater and lesser trochanters of the femur. Muscular actions pull the fracture proximally resulting in external rotation and shortening of the leg. This is a fracture of cancellous bone, and so the area has a good blood supply. The joint capsule is not generally involved. A fracture in this area does not usually interfere with the blood supply, and can usually be repaired without requiring a hip replacement. Surgical treatment of an inter-trochanteric fracture may involve open reduction, and fixation with a metal plate and screws. A metal rod down the center of the bone may be used in place of a plate. Physical therapy begins almost immediately, and healing time is about 12 weeks. This fracture often occurs due to a fall. Prognosis is excellent.

Pipkin Classification of Fractures

The Pipkin classification system is used to describe fractures of the femoral head. There are 4 types of Pipkin fracture. A Type I Pipkin fracture is a fracture of the head of the femur inferior to the fovea centralis with an associated posterior dislocation. A Type II Pipkin fracture is a fracture of the femoral head superior to the fovea centralis with an associated posterior dislocation. A Type III Pipkin fracture is a Type I, or II Pipkin fracture with an associated fracture of the femoral neck. A Type IV Pipkin fracture is a Type I, II, or III Pipkin fracture with an associated fracture of the acetabulum. Treatment depends upon the types of fracture and its severity.

Treatment for Femoral Head Fractures

Femoral neck fractures disconnect the head of the femur from the shaft of the femur. The blood supply is often interrupted at the time of fracture. The lack of an adequate blood supply impairs the healing process. This is especially true with a severe dislocation. For this reason, femoral fractures are often treated by a partial hip replacement. Treatment depends upon the severity of the dislocation, and the age of the patient. Hip replacements are usually performed in older, less active patients as they wear out with activity. A fractured femoral head with minimal displacement may treated by internal fixation. A partial hip replacement, or hip hemiarthroplasty, may be performed in which the head of the femur is replaced with a metal prosthesis. The prosthesis can be cemented onto the end of the bone, or press-fit. Rehabilitation is started right after surgery.

Garden Classification of Femoral Neck Fractures

The Garden classification covers fractures of the femoral neck. The basis of this classification is the displacement of the femoral head. There are 4 types. A Garden I fracture is an incomplete fracture of the femoral neck. It may be abducted, or impacted. This is a stable type of fracture. A Garden II fracture is a complete fracture of the femoral neck, but it is nondisplaced. This is also a stable fracture. A Garden III fracture is a complete fracture of the femoral neck with partial displacement. This fracture type may be stable, or unstable. A Garden IV fracture is a complete fracture of the femoral neck with complete displacement. This fracture type is unstable. Garden III fractures have a high risk for the development of avascular necrosis. The type of fracture affects treatment.

Gustilo and Anderson Classification of Open Fractures

There are 3 types, and 3 subtypes, of open fractures in the Gustilo and Anderson system. A Type I fracture refers to a fracture with an open wound of less than 1 centimeter. There is little damage to the muscle. The fracture involved is a simple fracture. A Type II fracture refers to a fracture with a wound greater than 1 centimeter in length with soft tissue damage. The fracture type is simple, or oblique with moderate comminution. A Type III fracture refers to a fracture with a wound that is greater than 1 centimeter in size involving extensive damage to the soft tissue. It involves damage to muscle, skin, and neurovascular structures. This is a high energy injury. A Type IIIA fracture has adequate soft tissue cover. A Type IIIB fracture has inadequate soft tissue cover with bone exposure. A Type IIIC fracture involves damage to an artery.

Danis-Weber Classification

The Danis-Weber classification system is used to describe ankle fractures. This system is based on the location of the fracture in relation to the syndesmosis, which is the sheath of tissue between the tibia and fibula. The syndesmosis is a ligament-like tissue. There are 3 types of Danis-Weber fracture. In a Type A fracture, the fracture is below the syndesmosis. In a Type B fracture the fracture is at the joint, level with the syndesmosis. The ligaments of the joint are usually not torn in this injury. This fracture may be associated with a fracture of the posterior part of the tibia. A Type C fracture is found above the syndesmosis. It may be associated with a tear of the deltoid ligament, an avulsion fracture of the tibia, and fractures of the malleolus.

Subcapital, Epicondylar, Supracondylar, and Transcondylar

A subcapital fracture is an intracapsular fracture at the site where the neck of the femur joins the head of the femur. It involves a fracture of the metaphysic, near the physis. An epicondylar fracture involves the epicondyles of the distal humerus. The epicondyles serve as attachment sites for muscles. Although lateral epicondylar fractures occur infrequently, medial epicondylar fractures are fairly common. A supracondylar fracture is a fracture located above the condyles, and epicondyles. This is the most common fracture in the region of the elbow. It is often difficult to diagnose. A transcondylar fracture is a transverse fractures across the condyles of the humerus, or femur. They often involve a fracture through the physis of the distal humerus.

Patella Fractures

Fractures of the patella commonly result from direct trauma to the anterior knee joint. Symptoms include severe pain, and instability of the knee. Examination of the extensor mechanism is vital with a suspected patella fracture. A careless examination, however, can displace a non-displaced fracture. The patient should be asked to lift the leg as a single unit 1-2 inches off of the exam table while the position of the lower leg in relation to the femur is assessed. The stability of the collateral ligaments of the knee with varus and valgus stressors must be tested. Since flexion of knee is contraindicated in patella fractures, an examination of the cruciate ligaments is not conducted. X ray studies are essential. A lateral x ray will help differentiate between displaced and non-displaced fractures. Non-displaced fractures can be treated with casting or a splint. Displaced fractures nearly always require open reduction and internal fixation.

Assessment of Possible Clavicle Fracture

Physical examination and radiographic studies are both important in assessment for a possible fracture of the clavicle. Clavicles are fractured frequently. A history of the injury should be taken. The patient should then disrobe to expose both clavicles and shoulders to allow visual inspection and comparison. Fractures of the clavicle sometimes press out, or "tent", the skin and this could result in skin damage allowing infection. A tenting clavicle fracture should be seen at once by the orthopedic surgeon. The clavicle should be palpated to determine the area of maximum tenderness. The sterno-clavicular, and acromio-clavicular joints should be examined for tenderness, or possible dislocation. An examination of the shoulder/glenohumeral joint should be conducted to determine that no concurrent injury has taken place. A clavicle fracture can result in injury to the neural and vascular structures near the fracture site.

Symptoms of Scaphoid Fracture

Fractures to the scaphoid bone (navicular bone) often result from falls on outstretched arms. Patients may present with radial sided wrist pain, significant swelling, and a limited range of motion in the wrist. To test for such fractures, palpate the area of the wrist just distal to the radial styloid in between the abductor pollicis longus, and the extensor pollicis longus tendons. This site is the anatomical snuff box. The scaphoid bone is found on the bottom of this area and will be painful on palpation if fractured. As a further test, grasp the metacarpal bone between the thumb and index fingers and gently push back towards the wrist. This may also produce pain in the case of a fractured scaphoid. Early scaphoid fractures do not always appear on radiographs; suspected scaphoid fractures should be treated with a thumb spica splint, or cast, until further diagnostic tests can be conducted.

Compartment Syndrome

The arms and legs are divided into several different compartments separated by connective tissue. Each compartment contains muscles as well as nerves and vascular structures. Abnormal pressure in a particular compartment can interfere with blood flow and perfusion to the structures within that compartment. This can lead to rapid irreversible damage to tissue if not addressed immediately. Compartment syndrome can result from a fracture if a large amount of blood collects in the compartment. Improper, or premature, casting can lead to compartment syndrome. If the affected extremity continues to swell, and the cast restricts the expansion, the muscles and nerves can become damaged. Bleeding into an extremity following surgery or traumatic laceration can quickly lead to compartment syndrome.

Tibial plateau fractures, femur fractures, and stab wounds of the extremities are risk factors for the development of compartment syndrome. Individuals with these injuries should be examined for signs of the disorder. Muscle ischemia is extremely painful. Pain out of proportion to the original injury is a symptom of compartment syndrome. On palpation, the affected extremity will feel full, and firm. Palpating the area will cause pain, as will passive movement of the extremity. The neurovascular status of the limb distal to the suspected compartment syndrome should be checked as an absent pulse, or disturbed sensation, is of great concern. Measurements of the compartment pressure can be performed with a special instrument, and readings approaching 30mmHG are of concern. Compartment syndrome is treated by surgical intervention to open the compartment and release the pressure.

Sprain and Strain

A sprain refers to an injury to a ligament. This can be as simple as a stretching of some of the fibers that make up the ligament to a complete tear of the entire ligament. These injuries are frequently graded I-III. Grade I sprains represent mild stretching of the ligament. Grade II sprains exhibit partial rupture, and Grade III sprains are complete ruptures. A strain is an injury to a muscle. This can be a stretching injury, or it can represent partial tearing of the muscle. Strains are accompanied by a state of inflammation in the affected muscular tissue. This injury is often seen in conjunction with a sprain when it occurs near the musculotendinous junction.

Dislocation

A dislocation occurs when a bone is separated from its articular surface. This injury is usually the result of trauma. There are a number of types of dislocation, and these are as follows: compound (open), complete, and incomplete (partial dislocation, or subluxation). A compound dislocation involves the total displacement of the bone from its articular surface together with skin damage so that the joint is exposed to the air. A complete dislocation involves the total separation of the bone from its articular surface which no damage to the skin. An incomplete fracture involves a displacement of the bone in which it is moved slightly out of its normal position. Treatment includes reduction, and perhaps immobilization. Surgery may be required to reduce a difficult dislocation, or to repair damaged tissue.

Meniscus Tear

The knee joint contains 2 cartilaginous disks called menisci that cushion and stabilize the knee joint. There is a lateral and medial meniscus in each knee located on the tibia, between the tibia and the femur. These menisci are crescent shaped with the opening of the crescent facing towards the middle of the knee joint. A tear of the meniscus is almost always painful. This pain is localized along the joint line. Often the pain from a torn meniscus radiates to the posterior portion of the knee. The pain may be constant, but likely increases when the patient weight bears, or pivots on the knee. With an acute meniscus tear, the knee joint will usually swell. Movement may produce a clicking sensation in the knee. Movement of the torn meniscus may cause the knee joint to lock. This could be intermittent in nature as the loose piece shifts around.

Joint Infection

Infection can affect any joint in the body, and this occurrence is a medical emergency. A complete physical assessment can determine if a joint is infected, or if the problem is simply a superficial skin infection. As a first step, the joint should be visually inspected. An infected joint will appear swollen, and the overlying skin may be red and irritated. The joint should be palpated. A joint that is noticeably warm to the touch, especially when compared with the uninvolved joint, is indicative of infection. The presence of fluid within the joint is a common finding with an infection. Active and passive range of motion should be assessed. An infected joint will be painful with any motion. If motion does not produce pain, then it is likely that the joint is not involved, and the infection is superficial.

Acute Rotator Cuff Tear

The rotator cuff is a complex of 4 muscles which work together to support the humeral head and function in shoulder motion. The most commonly injured muscle of the rotator cuff is the supraspinatus which helps to abduct the arm. Rotator cuff tears may result from an acute injury, but more frequently are the result of degenerative changes. Symptoms of an acute rotator cuff tear include pain in the shoulder which can radiate into the neck or arm, and difficulty with active abduction of the arm, especially past 90º. Tears may hamper the ability to smoothly lower the arm to the side after passive abduction. This is called a positive drop arm sign. Even a complete tear may not cause these symptoms in all patients, however. A strong deltoid muscle may compensate for the loss of the rotator cuff. Many conditions can mimic the symptoms of a rotator cuff tear.

Mallet Finger

Mallet finger is an injury to the extensor mechanism of the distal interphalangeal (DIP) joint. This injury can result from a forced flexion while the finger is extended. If the tendon of the extensor digitorum muscle is torn, this is called a soft tissue mallet finger. A bony mallet finger occurs when a small piece of bone from the distal phalanx is avulsed. An x ray is required to differentiate between these injuries. With either type of mallet finger, the patient's ability to actively extend the finger at the DIP joint is compromised. The patient will usually complain of a "droop" at the end of the finger. Palpation of the dorsal DIP joint will be tender in acute mallet finger injuries. The examiner should be able to passively extend the DIP joint without difficulty. If the finger cannot fully extend, the possibility of a displaced fracture needs to be considered.

Shoulder Adhesive Capsulitis

Adhesive capsulitis, or frozen shoulder, is a condition in which the soft tissues surrounding the shoulder become tight and restrictive. As a result, the range of motion of the affected shoulder is severely limited. Adhesive capsulitis can occur following an injury that causes the patient to hold the shoulder in limited motion for an extended period of time. Patients with diabetes can develop adhesive capsulitis without an injury or trauma. Physical examination of a patient with adhesive capsulitis will show a limited range of active and passive movement. The technologist must ensure that the patient does not affect the range of motion exam by leaning, or shrugging the shoulder to exaggerate motion. The treatment mainstay of adhesive capsulitis is aggressive physical therapy. Once the patient's range of motion is restored, a thorough physical examination may reveal the underlying injury.

Boutonniere Deformity

A boutonniere deformity is an injury to the central slip of the extensor mechanism over the proximal interphalangeal (PIP) joint. The extensor mechanism at this point of the finger is made up of three parts. The central portion, called the central slip, is in the midline and is flanked on each side by the dorsal expansions. If the central slip is ruptured, the phalanx is able to push through the void. This movement is driven by the dorsal expansions which move to the medial and lateral borders of the finger. The boutonniere deformity has a classic presentation. The affected finger will be fully flexed at the proximal interphalangeal joint. The distal interphalangeal and metacarpal phalangeal joints will be held in hyperextension.

Hip Trochanteric Bursitis

A bursa is a specialized structure in the body that allows tissue planes to move over one another smoothly. Bursitis occurs when the bursa become inflamed and the condition can be very painful. Bursitis can be caused by repetitive use. The bursa overlying the greater trochanter of the hip commonly becomes irritated and inflamed. Greater trochanteric bursitis will cause lateral hip pain that is worsened with direct pressure. The hip pain is often reported to spread distally along the lateral border of the thigh. Palpation of the greater trochanter in addition to hip rotation will reproduce the classic symptoms. It is always important to determine if there are any other sources of pain in a case of hip bursitis.

Hip Arthritis

Hip arthritis is a condition involving the loss of articular cartilage. The pain is frequently described as originating in the groin on the affected side. This is of importance in distinguishing hip pain from pain that originates in the lumbar spine which is usually felt posteriorly. The pain of hip arthritis is usually greatest when weight bearing, but also occurs at rest. Physical examination and x rays are used in diagnosis. The patient's gait is observed; the hip is palpated to determine if the patient is experiencing greater trochanteric bursitis which can mimic hip arthritis pain. The range of motion of the non-affected hip is tested first, and then compared to the painful hip. The degenerative changes of arthritis will restrict range of motion, and cause pain with flexion and rotation. An x ray examination is essential to determine the degree of degenerative change, and to rule out concurrent fracture.

Popliteal Cysts

A popliteal cyst, commonly referred to as a baker's cyst, is a collection of fluid in the posterior portion of the knee. This fluid is often an extension of the synovial fluid contained within the knee joint. Patients with a small popliteal cyst may present with a complaint of fullness in the popliteal space of the knee. A larger cyst may compress surrounding structures, causing pain and discomfort. Compression of neurovascular structures by a cyst can lead to pain radiating distally into the calf and foot. These cysts are usually palpable in the popliteal space however, they can fluctuate in size, and may be missed on physical examination. A popliteal cyst is usually the result of an underlying injury such as a meniscal tear, or a result of advanced degenerative changes. A physical examination should therefore be conducted to determine cause. The underlying cause should be treated.

Coxa Varum

Coxa varum is an abnormality of the hip which can be congenital, or acquired. It is the lateral (inward) turning of the hip. In this condition, the angle between the head and the shaft of the femur is abnormally decreased, being less than 120 degrees. Coxa varum may be caused by a traumatic injury, or it can result from a condition in which the bone tissue in the neck of the femur is abnormally soft. The bone then bends under the weight of the body. The abnormally soft bone can be congenital (Mau-Nilsonne Syndrome), or it may be due to a bone disorder. Coxa varum affects both hips in 25 – 50% of cases. The disorder causes pain, and results in difficulty in walking. An osteotomy can be performed to improve the condition.

Coxa Valga

Coxa valga is an abnormality of the hip which can be congenital or acquired. It is the medial (inward) turning of the hip joint. It is caused by a greater than normal angle (> 140 degrees) between the head and the shaft of the femur. This condition has to be diagnosed with the age of the patient in mind. At birth, the angle in question is approximately 150 degrees. This decreases gradually until the normal adult state is reached. Coxa valga is the persistence of the neonatal state, and is often the result of abductor muscle weakness, and a deficit in normal weight-bearing. Coxa valga is associated with numerous disorders including neuromuscular disorders, skeletal dysplasias, and juvenile idiopathic arthritis. If severe enough, the condition may result in the lateral subluxation, or dislocation of the head of the femur.

Genu Varum

Discuss Genu varum is an abnormality of the hip which can be congenital, or acquired. Inherited conditions, trauma, or disease can cause Genu varum. The disease is commonly known as bow-leggedness, or bandy-leg. In this condition, the knees are abnormally far apart, and the legs bow outwards. Generally, both the femur and tibia are curved outward. Many children go through a stage of being bow-legged, but the condition is usually outgrown. It may, however, persist. Persistent Genu varum may be caused by disease, such as rickets, or tibia vara (Blount's disease). Tibia vara is a deformity of the upper end of the tibia. In some cases, braces or surgery may be needed to correct Genu varum. Uncorrected, the condition may cause osteoarthritis.

Genu Valgum

Genu valgum is an abnormality of the hip which can be congenital, or acquired. The condition is commonly known as knock knees. The knees are in close association, and the feet are further apart than normal. The knees are in contact when the legs are straight, but the feet cannot be placed together. This condition is often seen in young children, but it usually corrects itself. If present in childhood, Genu valgum is usually resolved by puberty. The condition may persist, and worsen with increasing age. Genu valgum may result from a disease, such as rickets. It may result from obesity. Trauma can cause Genu valgum. Genu valgum may also be congenital. The congenital type is often idiopathic, meaning there is no known cause. Surgery may be used to correct Genu valgum.

Hallux Varus

Hallux Varus refers to the deviation of the big toe outward, toward the midline of the body. The condition can be congenital, or acquired. It is not uncommon to see this condition in children. The congenital condition is often due to a short abductor hallucis tendon, or a tight tendon. The condition can also result from trauma, some types of arthritis, removal of a sesamoid bone from the joint of the toe, and an unsuccessful bunion surgery. Treatment for this condition depends upon its severity. A mild condition may require no treatment. Stretching exercises and splinting may help.

Surgery may be indicated. Surgical possibilities include a tendon transfer. This is the reverse of a Hallux valgus.

Hallux Valgus

Hallux valgus refers to the deviation of the big toe inward away from the midline of the body. Although the head of the first metatarsal is turned medially, it may also be turned dorsally. Stress fractures may occasionally result from Hallux valgus. The sex ratio of this condition is 10:1 with more females being affected. Hallux valgus may be congenital in some cases, but can also be acquired. The condition may develop due to constricting shoes. This condition is painful, and can lead to deformity of the foot. The term Hallux valgus is not just another name for bunion. These are 2 separate conditions. A bunion, may, or may not, accompany Hallux valgus.

Bunions

A bunion is a bump on the inside of the big toe on the inner edge of the metatarsal. The bump can be a swollen bursal sac, a bony deformity, or both. The bunion may be associated with Hallux valgus. The condition is associated with the wearing of shoes. It affects more women than men. The physical effect of bunions varies dramatically. Some cause a great deal of pain and others do not. The degree of deformity is not necessarily linked to the amount of pain caused by the bunion. Treatment of a bunion may involve the wearing of a better fitting shoe, or surgery. Surgery may involve shaving off the bunion in conjunction with an osteotomy of the metatarsal.

Claw Toe

A claw toe involves the contraction of the toe at the middle and end joints (PIP and DIP). Tight ligaments and tendons cause the joint of the toe to curl downwards. The condition occurs in any toe but the big one. The top part of the toe rubs against the shoe, and the end of the toe that is tucked under presses against the insole of the shoe. There are 2 types of claw toes, and they are categorized according to the degree of flexibility of the joint involved. Claw toes are called either flexible or rigid depending upon whether or not the joint can be straightened manually. Claw toes can be congenital, or acquired. They may result from a muscular imbalance, or arthritis. Claw toes can also result from diseases that cause nerve damage, such as diabetes. Without treatment claw toe is progressive and permanent. Treatment includes splinting.

Hammer Toe

Hammer toe is a condition in which the second, third, or fourth toes are deformed by a bend at the middle joint. The injury is said to resemble a hammer. Although hammer toes are flexible at first, they can become fixed in their abnormal position. The condition causes pain in the toes, and sufferers may have difficulty finding shoes that are comfortable. The condition may cause corns or calluses on the affected toe. Hammer toe can be congenital, but can also be acquired. It may result from wearing shoes that are too short or an imbalance in the muscles. Although easily corrected in the early stages, it becomes more difficult as the condition worsens. Treatment varies with the severity of the condition. Treatment may include wearing roomier shoes, stretching exercises, and surgery if all else fails.

Mallet Toe

A mallet toe refers to the buckling of the joint (DIP joint) at the end of the toe. The affected toe develops a painful corn near the nail, and this corn may ulcerate. The other joint in the affected toe is normal. The second toe is the one most often affected by mallet toe. Mallet toe may be congenital or acquired. Mallet toe may occur when the toe is jammed, or it may result from wearing tight shoes. It may also result from a muscle imbalance or arthritis. An untreated mallet toe may result in permanent fixation of the joint. Treatment may include the recommendation to wear roomy shoes, exercises, or surgery. Surgery may involve cutting the tendons, internal fixation, or partial amputation.

Talipes

Talipes should be treated as early as possible in the child's life. Treatment must not only completely correct the deformity, but must ensure that it does not return. Early treatment for Talipes includes casting. This may be started at birth, and continue for several years. As the child is growing, the cast must be replaced every few weeks. Casting may be followed by several years of splinting, or bracing. These splints, or braces may need to be worn continually at first, at thereafter only at night. Physiotherapy may be successful in treating the disorder. Surgery may need to be performed to correct the disorder. The surgical technique depends upon the type of Talipes.

Talipes Valgus, Talipes Varus, Talipes Equines, and Talipes Calcaneus

These conditions are congenital deformities commonly referred to as clubfoot. The condition is caused by the abnormal development of the bones of the feet. The different types of Talipes represent different abnormalities of the foot. In all types of the condition, the feet are abnormally twisted. Talipes valgus involves the turning of the foot laterally, so the inside of the foot bears the weight. Talipes varus involves the turning of the foot medially, so that the outside of the foot bears the weight. Talipes equinus involves the downward pointing of the foot with the heel up. Talipes calcaneus involves the upward pointing of the foot with the heel down. Talipes can affect one or both feet. This condition does not resolve spontaneously, but requires medical intervention.

Ewing's Family of Tumors

Ewing's family of tumors (EFT) are malignant tumors that affect mostly adolescents and children. The tumors in this family all have the same characteristics. Although bones are most commonly affected, these tumors can be found in any tissue. It used to be thought that this tumor affected only bones, but now it is known that this is not the case. Ewing's tumors that affect different types of tissue have different names. Ewing's tumors affecting bone are usually found in the long bones, but other commonly affected sites are the pelvis and chest. The malignancy is thought to be caused by genetic mutations. Treatment may include chemotherapy, surgery, and radiation. The cure rate is fairly high.

Ganglion Cysts

A ganglion is a cystic growth that can develop anywhere on the wrist, or hand. It is not a malignant growth. A ganglion is a benign fluid-filled cyst. It develops from a joint capsule, or tendon sheath. What causes a ganglion to develop has not been determined. It has been theorized that these cysts result from damage to the tissue layer that produces synovial fluid. This fluid builds up outside its proper location in a joint of tendon, and forms an enlargement. Ganglions may cause pain, and changes in bone structure. Ganglions are attached their associated joint, or tendon sheath but not to the skin on top of them. Ganglions may resolve without treatment, or resolve with the immobilization of the affected area. Aspiration of the cysts may result in its permanent disappearance. Surgery may be indicated to excise the cyst. After excision, treatment involves a compression dressing, and splinting.

Osteosarcoma

Osteosarcoma, also called osteogenic sarcoma, is the most commonly occurring type of bone cancer in individuals under 20 years of age. The disease begins in the bones, and often metastasizes, particularly to the lungs. The disease occurs most frequently in the bones of the knee and upper arm. Osteosarcoma affects more boys than girls, and occurs more often in black children than in white children. It begins most often during the growth spurt of adolescence, because the affected bone cells are osteoblasts. These are the cells that form bone. Individuals who had radiation therapy in childhood are more likely to develop the disease then those who did not. There does seem to be a genetic component to this cancer. Pain, swelling and fractures are symptoms of osteosarcoma. Surgery, chemotherapy, and radiation are used to treat the cancer. The survival rate at five years is 65 percent.

Multiple Myeloma

Multiple myeloma, also commonly called plasma cell myeloma, is a cancer of the plasma cells. Multiple myeloma is classified as a hematological malignancy. Plasma cells comprise part of the body's immune system. They are found in bone marrow. The cancer cells eventually build up in the bone resulting in its destruction. Multiple myeloma may cause bone pain, particularly in the vertebral column, and in the ribs. It can also cause broken bones. The cause of this cancer is not known. Treatment generally involves chemotherapy, or radiation. Stem cell transplantation may be a possibility. Multiple myeloma is difficult to treat, and relapse often follows treatment. The prognosis is generally very poor. Treatment is often palliative.

Osteoma

An osteoma is a nonmalignant mass of new bone. These tumors develop mostly on the bones of the skull and face, but may also be found on the clavicle, pelvic bones, and tubular bones. There are also soft tissue osteomas, and these occur usually in the eye and tongue. Osteomas may be associated with pain at the site of the tumor which increases at night, and with activity. Osteomas generally develop in late childhood, or early adulthood. They are slow growing tumors which are benign, and do not become malignant. Osteomas may disappear spontaneously. Osteomas may produce no symptoms, and if asymptomatic, no treatment is necessary. Treatment, if necessary, is by excision.

Chondroma

Chondroma is a noncancerous tumor formed of cartilage. It is thought to originate in epiphyseal cartilage. This benign tumor generally develops in the bones of the hands or feet, but it also develops in the long bones, and ribs. These tumors can occur in several types of tissue, and are categorized according to the tissue in which they are found. The types of chondroma are as follows: enchondroma, periosteal chondroma, and soft tissue chondroma. These tumors develop in bone, on the surface of bone, and in soft tissue respectively. This tumor doesn't usually produce symptoms, but occasionally causes pain at the site of the tumor. If the tumor produces no symptoms, treatment is not usually necessary. Treatment is excision.

Synovial Osteochondromatosis

Synovial osteochondromatosis (SOC) is a condition in which the joint is filled with multiple loose fragments. These loose fragments are made of cartilage or bone. These loose fragments are called joint mice. There are two types of the disorder: familial, and non-familial. The familial type occurs early in life and involves numerous very small particles. The non-familial type presents later in life, and involves particles of different sizes. SOC can affect any synovial joint, but usually affects the knee, hip, elbow, and shoulder. The condition is nonmalignant, but results in joint degeneration and arthritis. The constant irritation of the fragments irritates the joint and causes the production of excess synovial fluid. The joint mice may cause the joint to lock, if they become trapped between the articulating surfaces.

Giant Cell Tumor

A giant cell tumor is a fast growing benign bone tumor which develops in the long-bones. This condition is rare, and is generally seen in individuals 20 to 40 years of age. They are called giant cell tumors as they are the result of the merging of several normal cells. Large complex tumor cells are formed in this way. These tumors occur most commonly in the distal femur, or proximal tibia. They also occur in the wrist and the hip. These tumors produce pain in the bone, and swelling. The pain decreases with rest, and increases with activity. It also gets progressively worse as the tumor enlarges. The cause of giant cell tumor is not known. It does not seem to be hereditary, and seems to develop spontaneously. Trauma does not appear to be a cause. These tumors destroy bone, and must be treated. Treatment involves surgery and bone grafting.

Bucket Handle Tear

A bucket handle tear is a particular type of meniscal tear. This type of meniscal tear results from trauma. It is seen inn younger and older patients, but it is not the result of degenerative processes. In this injury, the meniscus is torn around the rim. The middle part of the torn meniscus, which resembles a bucket handle, may become wedged in the joint. Although bucket handle tears may occur in both the medial and lateral menisci, they occur most often in the medial meniscus. This type of meniscal tear interferes with normal functioning of the knee, which cannot be fully extended. This phenomenon is known as locking. Treatment may involve arthroscopic surgery to remove the fragment of meniscus.

Internal Derangement of the Knee Joint

Internal derangement of the knee joint is a chronic condition involving a disruption in the inner structure of the joint. This condition interferes with normal function and activities. This term covers a number of abnormalities in the structure of the knee joint. Any of the following structures may be involved: the collateral ligaments, cruciate ligaments, and semilunar cartilages (menisci). The most common internal derangement of the knee joint involves damage to the medial collateral ligament. The medial meniscus, and the anterior cruciate ligament or the next most frequently affected. Symptoms depend upon the severity of the injury. Pain and swelling are common. Functional impairment occurs to varying degrees depending upon the structure injured, and the extent of damage. Treatment involves diagnosis and repair by arthroscopy, and arthroscopic surgery. Prognosis depends upon the actual injury.

Osteoarthritis

Osteoarthritis, also called degenerative arthritis, is the most common arthritic disorder. It occurs when the articular cartilage degenerates. In the first stages, pieces of cartilage may break off and cause pain. Bone spurs may appear where the bones contact each other. The joint may be difficult to move. The cartilage may eventually erode completely, allowing the ends of the bones to rub together. Swelling of the joint may occur at this stage. Osteoarthritis may have other adverse effects as the joint is used less due to pain. The muscles may weaken, and the joint may become distorted. This disorder generally affects the hips, knees, hands and vertebral column. Any joint may be affected, however. The cause of osteoarthritis is unknown, but the disorder affects men and women equally. It generally occurs after the age of 45. Heredity, excess weight, injury, overuse, and other types of arthritis are risk factors.

Osteoarthritis is diagnosed by physical examination, blood tests, joint fluid tests, and imaging tests. The disease cannot be cured, but most forms can be managed. Non-prescription analgesics are a mainstay of treatment. Non-prescription topical gels and creams may provide some relief. Codeine or nonsteroidal anti-inflammatories (NSAIDS) may be prescribed for pain management. None of these treatments will prevent further damage. Corticosteroids may be injected into the affected joint, but this treatment may damage bones and cartilage if given too often. Low impact exercises may be recommended to strengthen the joint, but these will not prevent further damage from the condition. A new treatment called viscosupplementation may be recommended. In this treatment, a gel is injected into the joint to lubricate it allowing easier movement. Surgery may be indicated. This can range from cleaning the debris from the joint, to joint replacement.

Dupuytren's Disease

Dupuytren's disease is a condition which involves the shrinking and thickening of the fascia under the skin of the palm of the hand. Dupuytren's disease distorts the normal hand position. The shrinking of the fascia forces the fingers into a bent position. It also causes bumps and depressions in the skin covering the palm of the hand. The disease affects the ring finger and pinky more than the other fingers, but they all may be affected. The severity of the disease varies among affected individuals. It is a progressive disease. There seems to be an inherited component to the disorder, which appears in adulthood. Individuals of northern European descent are at highest risk of developing the disease. Trauma is not involved. Surgery is the normal treatment, and produces good results. The disease can recur, however.

Rheumatoid Arthritis

Rheumatoid arthritis is classed as an autoimmune disease. It causes severe pain, inflammation, and distorted joints. An autoimmune disease is one in which the body launches an attack against its natural antibodies because it mistakenly perceives these as being foreign. During this disease process, the body produces another kind of antibody, called rheumatoid factors (RF), to fight the normal antibodies. The first stage of the disease is synovitis, which is inflammation of the synovial tissues. The disease is progressive, and eventually leads to the immobility of the joint, or joints. The inflammation associated with this disease is caused by an inflammatory substance called pannus which is secreted by the RF antibodies. The pannus sticks to the joint surfaces damaging cartilage and bone, and causing stiffness. This stiffness is known as ankylosis. Osteoarthritis can result in a permanent deformity in the affected joint or joints. The hands and feet are most commonly affected. Rheumatoid arthritis can also affect the organs.

Rheumatoid arthritis most commonly affects individuals between the ages of 25 and 50, but it is seen in all age groups. If diagnosed early, the disease can be controlled, and damage lessened. The disease is diagnosed by x-ray, blood tests, and joint fluid tests. NSAIDS reduce pain and swelling, but not damage to the joints. Disease-modifying anti-rheumatic drugs (DMARDS) may be prescribed to prevent rheumatoid arthritis from progressing. The action of this family of drugs is to slow or stop the progression of the disease by suppressing the immune reaction. They cannot repair damage already done. For some patients, gold injections are effective in lessening the effects of the disease. Corticosteroids and biologics may be prescribed. Biologics block hormones that are involved in causing inflammation. Surgery, ranging from the removal of damaged tissue to joint replacement may be beneficial.

Psoriatic Arthritis

Psoriatic arthritis is also called arthropathic psoriasis. The condition is classified as a seronegative spondyloarthropathy. It is an autoimmune disease. This inflammatory arthritis is associated with psoriasis. Approximately 20% of individuals with psoriasis are also affected with psoriatic arthritis, and the symptoms of the arthritis appear about 10 years after the appearance of the psoriasis. Occasionally the symptoms of arthritis will precede those of the psoriasis. Symptoms of this type of arthritis include nail lesions, and loss of the nails. Psoriatic arthritis can also cause tendonitis, and dactilytis. Dactilytis is a swelling of the joints. On x-ray, the affected areas look fluffy. There are 5 main types of this condition. These are as follows: symmetric, asymmetric, arthritis mutilans, spondylitis, and distal interphalangeal predominant.

Symmetric psoriatic arthritis is the most common type, accounting for 50% of all cases. It affects both sides of the body at the same time. The Asymmetric type is the next most common type, affecting 35% of psoriatic arthritis sufferers. It is a milder form of the condition. It occurs on only 1 side of the body, and involves fewer joints. Arthritis mutilans is much rarer, and much more severe. It is a progressive disease, and deforms and destroys the joints over time. Spondylitis generally affects the spinal column, causing stiffness, but it can also occur in the hands and feet. The distal interphalangeal predominant type causes inflammation of the joints at the ends of the digits. It causes obvious changes in the nails.

Psoriatic arthritis is diagnosed by means of blood tests, x-rays, and joint fluid tests. The erythrocyte sedimentation rate can be used in diagnosis. An increased rate of sedimentation indicates psoriatic arthritis. Blood tests can determine if the rheumatoid factor, which is an antibody for rheumatoid arthritis, is present. This antibody is not present in psoriatic arthritis, and its presence can be used to differentiate between the diseases. Psoriatic arthritis may be treated with anti-inflammatory drugs, corticosteroid joint injections, immunosuppressants, and antirheumatic drugs. Corticosteroid inject is not practical if the joints are widely affected. Immunosuppressant drugs also treat the psoriasis. Treatment recommendations may include tumor necrosis factor inhibitors. This class of biologic drugs has been developed recently, and may prevent irreversible damage to the joints.

Ankylosing Spondylitis

Ankylosing spondylitis is a type of spondylarthropathy, which is a group of diseases that affect the spine. Ankylosing spondylitis has a very variable presentation, and the course of the disease varies among individuals. Some individuals with the disorder have intermittent back pain, while other individuals have severe and ongoing pain that leads to stiffness of the vertebral column. Between episodes, the disease course includes periods of remission. In addition to pain in the spine, individuals with the disorder may experience pain in the other parts of the body, including the ribs, shoulders, and hips. The disease may also cause eye inflammation, blurry vision, and pain. The back pain caused by the disease has been described as dull and diffuse. The affected individual may adopt a bent over posture to ease the pain. If the disease is not treated, bony outgrowths may develop on the vertebra, interfering with motion and function.

Ankylosing spondylitis is also called simply spondylitis is a chronic inflammatory arthritis of the vertebral column. The disease is crippling, and causing pain, and affecting posture. Individuals with this disease are force to adopt a bent over position. Ankylosing spondylitis occurs as a result of inflammation which can eventually worsen to the point that the vertebrae fuse. Fusion of the vertebrae severely restricts movement. The disease particularly damages the sacroiliac joint which is where the spine joins the pelvis. The disease typically strikes young people between the ages of 15 and 30. It can affect individuals at a younger age, but the disease usually has a different presentation in these cases. Younger individuals affected with spondylitis usually experience pain in the joints of the lower limbs before the disease moves into the spine. It is very rare for this disease to appear in individuals after the age of 40.

Ankylosing spondylitis cannot be cured. There are treatments to control pain, and limit the damage done by the disease. Early treatment is essential. X-rays taken in the early stages may not show arthritic changes. It takes time for these to develop. Arthritic changes will eventually be evident in the sacroiliac joint, and edges of some vertebrae.

There is not blood test for the diagnosis of ankylosing spondylitis, but the erythrocyte sedimentation test can tell if inflammation is present. Stiffness of the spine is diagnostic. Treatment includes NSAIDS and corticosteroids to reduce inflammation, and disease-modifying anti-rheumatic drugs (DMARDS) to prevent further damage to the joints. Biologics may be prescribed to block the inflammatory effects of hormones Exercise will help keep the joints mobile, but certain exercise may increase the risk of fracture. Damaged joints may require surgical replacement. The hip is the joint most commonly replaced. Prognosis is variable.

Spondylosis

Spondylosis is a type of osteoarthritis of the spine. The disease is degenerative. It damages the structure of the vertebral column, and interferes with its function. It is a disease of aging, but the course of the disease is variable and individual. The cervical, thoracic, and lumbar divisions of the vertebral column are affected. The intervertebral disks, facet joints, bones and ligaments of the vertebral column may be affected, and show degenerative changes.

Cervical spondylosis causes neck pain which may radiate into the shoulder. Thoracic spondylosis can cause pain on flexion, and hyperextension. Spondylosis of the lumbar region can cause pain with sitting for extended periods of time, or activities requiring repetitive bending.

Palpation of the spinal column may reveal structural abnormalities, and areas of soreness. A range of motion test determines the extent of the ability to flex, extend, laterally bend, and rotate the spinal joints. Imaging tests can look for structural problems. A neurological examination can determine if there are any sensory, or motor, deficits. The pain of cervical spondylosis may be relieved by wearing a cervical collar which supports the neck, and keeps the vertebrae separated. Continual use of a cervical collar can weaken the muscles of the neck, however, and is not recommended. Physiotherapy and NSAIDS can ease pain. Injection of the spinal joints may help control pain. Surgery to fuse vertebrae, or to remove parts of a disk, may be indicated. In a fusion, bones from the hip are removed and attached to 2 vertebrae by screws. This prevents dislocation of the joint.

Spondylolysis

Spondylolysis, sometimes called pars defect, is a condition which involves a fracture of the pars interarticularis. The pars interarticularis is the bony ring of the back of a vertebra. This ring is the weakest section of the vertebra. Spondylolysis is generally the result of strain. It occurs when the spinal column is bent backwards repeatedly. The fracture can occur at any age, but it occurs most often in children and adolescents because their vertebral columns are in the process of maturing. Symptoms of this fracture cause pain and stiffness in the lower back. The pain may radiate down the legs because of pressure on the nerves resulting from the fracture. This is called neurogenic pain. This occurs because extra cartilage is formed as a part of the healing process, and this can press on the nerve. This pressure can produce tingling in the legs, and cause pain and weakness.

Diagnostics tools include X-rays, and bone scans. The Scotty dog sign is indicative of spondylolysis. On x-ray, the outline of the vertebra normally looks like a dog. If spondylolysis is present, there is a small crack across the neck of the dog which has been likened to a collar. As a small crack may not be evident on x-ray a CT scan, or MRI is often conducted. Spondylolysis often heals itself with rest. A back brace, or cast for 3 – 4 months may be necessary. Surgery is not usually required, but if symptoms do not abate it may be necessary. Surgical procedures include laminectomy, and posterior lumbar fusion. A laminectomy is the removal of the lamina from the ars interarticularis. This is performed to relieve pressure on the nerve. A fusion may be performed after a laminectomy, or to stabilize the spinal segment.

Spondylolisthesis

Spondylolisthesis is a condition where 1 vertebra slides forward in the vertebral column. It may be caused by spondylolysis. Spondylolisthesis usually involves a vertebra in the lumbar region. Symptoms of this condition may include one or more of the following: pain in the lumbar region, thighs, or legs; muscle spasms; and weakness in the lumbar region. Symptoms vary in severity among affected individuals. Mild cases may show no symptoms. Individuals with a severe case may look swayback, and waddle. The condition may be congenital, or acquired. A congenitally thin bone in the vertebra may predispose an individual to developing the condition. The condition may also result from physical stress, and trauma. The spine itself can be compromised as the damage to the vertebrae progresses

The Wiltse classification system lists 5 types of spondylolisthesis. These are as follows: dysplastic, isthmus, degenerative, traumatic, and pathologic. Dysplastic spondylolisthesis is occurs due to a congenital defect of the lumbrosacral junction. This is a rare form of the condition. It is progressive, and causes neurological problems. Prognosis is poor, and treatment is difficult because of the poorly developed vertebra. Isthmic spondylolisthesis is the most frequently observed form of the disorder. The condition is not usually progressive. The condition is often asymptomatic. Degenerative spondylolisthesis is the result of arthritis, and bone remodeling. It occurs in individuals over the age of 50. In this case, the spondylolisthesis can produce spinal stenosis. Traumatic spondylolisthesis is extremely uncommon. It may occur due to severe fracture of the bony ring of the spine. Pathologic spondylolisthesis is extremely rare. It is associated with cancer, metabolic bone disease, tumors, tuberculosis, and Paget's disease of bone.

Meyerding Grading System

The Meyerding system grades the severity of the vertebral slip of spondylolisthesis. It is used to describe all types of spondylolisthesis. It is based on measurements of the distance between the posterior edge of one vertebra to the posterior edge of the vertebra immediately underneath. This measurement is then expressed as a percentage of the height of the superior vertebra. The measurements are obtained from x-rays. There are 4 grades, and these are as follows from a low level of slippage to high: Grade 1 (0 -25%), Grade 2 (25 – 50%), Grade 3 (50 – 75%), and Grade 4 (75 – 100%). A ranking of over 100% indicates that the upper vertebra slides off the lower vertebra completely. Spondyloptosis is the term used to describe a situation of complete slippage.

Treatment

Spondylolisthesis is diagnosed by lateral x-ray. Treatment depends upon the type and grade of the condition. If the case is asymptomatic, and stable, no treatment is necessary. In these cases, the condition should be monitored. If the condition is painful and progressing, treatment is necessary. Activities that place stress on the area should be avoided. Medications may be prescribed for pain. Corsets and braces may be advised to provide support. Surgery may be indicated if more conservative measures fail to relieve symptoms. The goal of surgery is to relieve pressure on the nerves of the spine, and to stabilize the spine. Surgery involves reduction, and fusion of the affected joint. Depending upon the site of injury, surgery can be performed from the front of the vertebral column, or the back.

CES

Cauda equine syndrome (CES) is a condition affecting the nerve roots housed in the end of the spinal column. This condition constitutes a medical emergency. In CES, the nerves roots become compressed interfering with sensory and motor functions. Left untreated, CES may lead to such problems as permanent paralysis, permanently impaired bladder control, permanently impaired bowel control, and sexual dysfunction. Even with prompt treatment, deficits in these areas may result. There are many possible causes of CES including stenosis of the spinal canal, tumor, infection, a damaged spinal disk, and trauma. CES can also be congenital. The condition may cause a loss of sensation in the buttocks and lower extremities. This may be progressive. MRI and CT are used in diagnosis. Surgery is necessary to correct the problem. The type of surgery depends upon the cause. Surgery will not correct nerve damage, but may prevent further damage.

Paget's Disease of Bone

Paget's disease of bone is also called osteitis deformans. It is a chronic disorder of the bone and involves a disturbance in the normal rates of breakdown and build up of bone. The disease shows up most often in the spine, skull, pelvis and legs. Paget's disease of bone may cause hearing impairment if it affects the skull. In Paget's disease, these 2 processes occur much more quickly than normal. The disease results in weak and deformed bones. Paget's disease can lead to pain, fractures, arthritis, and deformities of the skeleton. The disease appears to have a hereditary component. It is also thought to be caused by a slow acting viral infection. Paget's disease is generally diagnosed in those over 40 years of age. More men are affected than women.

Diagnostic methods include radiographs, and bone scans. Blood tests of those with Paget's disease of the bone may show an elevated level of alkaline phosphatase. The course of the disease is slow, and it does not spread to healthy bone. Although there is no cure for Paget's disease of the bone, it can be controlled. Drug treatment is aimed at controlling pain, and slowing the progression of the disease. There are specific drugs to treat Paget's disease of bone. Surgery may be needed to correct damage caused by the disease. The surgical procedures may involve cutting and resetting the bone, and joint replacement. Surgery may also be used to aid in fracture healing. Calcium supplements should be a part of the diet. NSAIDS can relieve pain, but do not prevent damage to the skeletal system.

Boutonnière Deformity

Boutonnière deformity can result from acute trauma, burns, infections, and arthritis. Trauma, burns, and infectious processes may damage the central slip. Rheumatoid arthritis causes chronic inflammation of synovial tissue. This inflammation may force the PIP into a flexed position, stretching the central slip and causing its rupture. This in turn may increase tension on the DIP extensors resulting in hyperextension of the DIP. There are 3 degrees of boutonnière deformity caused by rheumatoid arthritis. These are mild (Stage I), moderate (Stage II) and severe (Stage III). A Stage I condition can be treated with splinting. A Stage II case requires surgery. Treatment depends upon the severity of the condition. Prognosis is good for Stage I and Stage II cases stemming from rheumatoid arthritis, and in cases of acute trauma. Other cases do not respond as well to treatment. Salvage procedures may be needed. Amputation is a last resort.

Erosive Osteoarthritis

Erosive osteoarthritis, also called inflammatory osteoarthritis, is the most common form of osteoarthritis. The disease is strongly hereditary. The disease is found most often in white females over the age of 60. Although this time coincides with menopause, not link to hormone levels has been found. The symptoms of the disease include swelling and pain in the finger joints, along with cyst formation. There may be a misalignment in the affected joints. Erosive osteoarthritis can be diagnosed by x-ray. Blood tests are not generally useful in diagnosis, as the result are usually normal no matter how severe the disease. Treatment may involve occasional splinting to prevent joint deformity, NSAIDS, and corticosteroid injections. Reconstructive surgery may be needed. The joints may be surgically fused.

Swan-Neck Deformity

Swan-neck deformity is a common deformity of the metacarpophalangeal (MP), proximal interphalangeal (PIP), and distal interphalangeal (DIP) joints in individuals with rheumatoid arthritis. The deformity occurs as a result of inflammation of the synovial tissue. This inflammation disturbs the interaction between the flexors and extensors of the joints. Nalebuff described 4 categories of swan-neck deformities. These are as follows: Type I, where the PIP joint is flexible, and can move in every direction; Type II, where the ability of the PIP joint to flex is limited in some positions; Type III where the ability of the PIP joint to flex is limited in all directions; and Type IV, where the PIP joint is completely inflexible, and appears damaged in imaging studies.

Type I Swan-Neck Deformity

A Type I swan-neck deformity can occur at the proximal phalangeal joint, or the distal phalangeal joint. Damage to either one of these joints can cause the classic manifestation of this condition. The classic appearance of swan-neck involves hyperextension at the PIP joint, and flexion at the DIP joint. In this type of swan-neck deformity the PIP joint can still be actively flexed. A PIP joint involvement is caused by inflammation of the synovial tissue, or a rupture of the, flexor digitorum superficialis tendon resulting in the stretching of the joint capsule. A DIP involvement begins with damage to the terminal tendon attachment at the distal phalanx of the muscles involved in extension. This results in an imbalance of muscle action leading to an increased stress on the central slip. This, along with slackness in the volar plate of the PIP joint leads to hyperextension at the PIP joint.

Nalebuff's Classification

Nalebuff classifies swan-neck deformities into the following 4 types:

- Type I - PIP joints are flexible in all positions.
- Type II - PIP joint flexion is limited in certain positions.
- Type III - PIP joint flexion is limited in all positions.
- Type IV - PIP joints are stiff and have a poor radiographic appearance.

Treatment

Type I swan-neck deformities can be treated by splinting. The goal is to allow the PIP joint to flex while preventing the hyperextension of the joint. A Type II swan-neck deformity is treated by relieving the constriction of the joint by a surgical release. A Type III swan-neck deformity is treated by surgical reconstruction, the goal of which is to return the ability to flex to the PIP joint. A Type IV swan-neck deformity is treated with a salvage-type surgical procedure. This involves an arthrodesis (fusion of the joint), or arthroplasty depending upon the severity and site of the damage. Fusion is often used to treat the index, and middle fingers to ensure lateral stability. Arthroplasty (joint replacement) is often recommended for the ring and pinky fingers to allow the retention of the ability to grasp.

Trigger Finger

Trigger finger involves damage to the tendons that aid in bending the fingers and thumb. It is classified as a stenosing tenosynovitis. This is a condition in which the sheath surrounding a tendon becomes inflamed and swollen, or when a nodule forms on a tendon; this prevents the tendon from moving freely in the sheath. The digit involved can be bent, but is difficult and painful to straighten. A popping, or cracking noise may be heard when the finger is straightened. All digits may be affected. This injury is seen most commonly in individuals between 40 and 60 years of age. It occurs more often in individuals with diabetes, and rheumatoid arthritis. Splinting may allow this injury to heal. Corticosteroid injects may ease the pain. Surgery may be useful to stop permanent stiffness from developing. This involves opening the tunnel of the tendon sheath.

Gamekeeper's Thumb

Gamekeeper's thumb is an injury to the ulnar ligament at the joint of the thumb and palm. It is also called a skiers thumb, or UCL tear. It was originally called gamekeeper's thumb because this injury used to be common in gamekeepers due to their technique of carrying, or killing, game. The injury is the result of forceful abduction of the thumb. It is also called skiers thumb because this injury is often sustained during a fall when the thumb gets caught in the ski pole loop. The injury involves the stretching, or tearing of the ligament away from the bone. A small chip of bone may also be avulsed. Treatment may involve casting, splinting, or surgery to reattach the ligament. The ligament may be reattached to the bone with an anchor. Surgery should be performed as soon as possible for best results. Arthritis may result from this injury.

Ulnar Nerve Entrapment

Ulnar nerve entrapment involves the compression of the nerve running from the collarbone down the inside of the arm. This is the ulnar nerve. Ulnar nerve entrapment interferes with the normal functioning of the arm. Entrapment of the nerve results in a numb feeling in the ring finger, and pinky. The use of the fingers is impaired, and the inside of the elbow may ache. These symptoms occur most often when the elbow is bent. As the nerve travels down the arm, it passes through the cubital tunnel which is found behind the inner part of the elbow. The nerve then proceeds down the arm and into the hand. Once in the hand, the nerve passes through Guyon's canal. The most likely site of compression is in the back of the elbow, but compression of the nerve at the wrist and near the neck also occurs.

Fractures of the elbow, bone spurs, cysts, and trauma are risk factors for development of ulnar nerve entrapment. The site of entrapment may provide a clue as to the cause of the condition. Symptoms of the condition include numbness in the ring finger and pinky finger, muscle weakness, coordination problems in the hand, and muscle wasting. If muscle wasting should occur, it is irreversible. A physical examination is used to diagnose the problem. This might involve manipulation of the joints in the affected extremity to determine symptoms of the condition can be elicited. X-rays may be taken to look for bone spurs. A nerve conduction test, to see how well nerve impulses are transmitted down the arm may be conducted. The patient may be advised simply to avoid movements that constrict the nerve. Anti-inflammatory drugs may be prescribed, as well as steroid injections.

In the case of a severe problem that does not improve with non-surgical treatments surgery may be advised. The exact type of surgery depends upon the area of compression. The most common compression sit is the elbow, and therefore this is the most common surgical site. Surgery may be performed at the wrist, or at the wrist and elbow if necessary. Surgery around the elbow may involve cutting cubital tunnel. It may also involve the relocation of the nerve from its place behind the elbow to a place in front of the elbow. This procedure is known as an anterior transposition of the ulnar nerve. The nerve may also be moved to several other sites. These surgeries are called subcutaneous transposition, submuscular transposition and intermuscular transposition. If the location of compression is at the wrist, the top of Guyon's canal will be cut. Any existing cysts will be removed.

Enchondroma

Enchondromas are nonmalignant tumors of the bone that being developing in the cartilage. Enchondroma generally develops in the cartilage lining the insides of bones. It most often affects the long bones of the hands and feet, but may also affect the other log bones of the body. An enchondroma is the most commonly seen tumor of the hand. The tumor is seen most often in young individuals between the ages of 10 and 20. The cause of enchondroma is uncertain. It may result from the persistence of embryonic cartilage, or it may simply be an overgrowth of cartilage. Enchondroma may cause pain, and may lead to bone fractures. It can deform the bone. It may also be asymptomatic. Enchondroma may involve a single tumor, or multiple tumors. Ollier's disease, also called enchondromatosis, and Maffucci's syndrome are both diseases involving multiple enchondromas. These diseases can cause deformity.

An enchondroma is often found during a routine physical examination. It may also be found during x-rays taken for reasons of fracture, or arthritis. Pain from the tumor may prompt x-rays of the bone. Diagnostic tests include x-rays, and bone scans. It is important to determine whether any tumor is benign or malignant. In x-ray, enchondromas look small and white. The enchondroma will contain arcs that mark it as containing cartilage. Asymptomatic enchondroma may just be watched to ensure it is not growing. Treatment may include surgery, where the tumor is excised, and the hole filled with a bone graft. If a fracture has occurred due to the enchondroma, it is allowed to heal, and then the tumor is excised.

Chondrosarcoma

Chondrosarcoma is a type of cancer of the bone that forms in cartilaginous cells. It is a primary bone cancer, meaning it begins in the bone rather than beginning in another tissue and traveling to the bone. The bones of the extremities and spine are most often affected. Other bones are affected, but less frequently. Chondrosarcoma is rare individuals under the age of 20. It is most common in individuals between 50 and 70 years of age. The disease affects males and females in equal numbers. The aggressiveness of this cancer, meaning its speed of growth and the ease with which it spreads, is rated on a scale of 1 – 4. A grade 1 cancer is slow growing and a Grade 4 cancer is extremely aggressive. A bone fracture may be the first sign that the cancer is present.

Diagnostic methods include biopsy, x-ray, and bone scans (CT and MRI). Chondrosarcoma may evolve from a number of conditions involving cartilaginous tumors, but the disease usually originates in normal cartilage cells. The primary and most successful treatment for this cancer is surgery. Chemotherapy and radiation therapy are not very effective in treating chondrosarcoma. Proton therapy has shown some success in treating this cancer. Amputation of the affected bone may be necessary. If the cancer is located in an area that makes full ablation difficult, or impossible, proton therapy may be a useful supplementary treatment. Chemotherapy may also be used for this purpose. Follow-up care involving bones scans are essential as this cancer recur easily.

Olecranon Bursitis

Olecranon bursitis is commonly known as elbow bursitis, or Popeye elbow). In this condition, fluid collects in the bursa behind the elbow. The bursa normally allows smooth, painless motion of the elbow joint. When the olecranon bursa becomes inflamed, it causes pain in the elbow. Bursitis of the elbow may arise from trauma. It may also without any apparent reason. The condition may be made worse by the habit of resting weight on the elbows. Swelling and pain in the back of the joint are symptoms. Inflammation of the bursa can also result from an infection, and this is a much more serious condition called infected elbow bursitis. Individuals with gout and rheumatoid arthritis are more likely to develop infected elbow bursitis than are members of the general population. Symptoms of an infected bursa in the elbow are elevated temperature, chills, sweating, localized redness, and localized skin damage.

Lipoma

A lipoma is a nonmalignant tumor which develops from fatty tissue. These tumors are soft, and usually cause no pain. They are slow growing, but may grow to be large than 6 centimeters. Lipomas occur most often in adults, but do occur in children. They are quite common, occurring in 1 out of 100 people. There are 5 types of lipoma which are named according to the type of tissue in which they occur. These are as follows: superficial subcutaneous, intramuscular, spindle cell, angiolipoma, and other. The "other" category includes lipomas occurring in other types of tissue such as the tendon sheath, nerves, or synovium. The superficial subcutaneous type is the most commonly occurring. The cause of this tumor is unknown. Removal of a lipoma may be by excision, or liposuction. The tumor may regrow if the capsule is not completely removed. Lipomatosis is a condition involving multiple lipomas.

Lymphedema

Lymphedema (lymphoedema) is also called lymphatic obstruction. It involves fluid retention in a specific part of the body caused by a poorly functioning lymphatic system. The lymphatic system is in charge of collecting, circulating, and filtering the interstitial fluid of the body. Lymphedema can lead to infection in the affected limb. The condition can be inherited (primary lymphedema), or acquired (secondary lymphedema) through damage to the lymphatic vessels. The condition is often seen as an aftermath of lymph node removal, or surgery which damages the lymphatic system. Radiation therapy can also cause this condition by damaging the lymphatic system. It is common in women after breast cancer surgery, where the upper body is affected. Any surgery that involves the removal of lymph nodes can cause the condition. Some parasitic infections will cause secondary lymphedema.

Staging

Lymphedema progresses in 4 set stages, 0 - 3. Stage 0 is the latent stage. Although the lymphatic system has been damaged, the damage has yet to become evident. Circulation is still adequate, and fluid has not begun to accumulate. Stage 1 is the spontaneously reversible stage. In Stage 1, fluid accumulation is just beginning. The affected area is normal, or near normal in appearance. The affected region indents and rebounds appropriately when pressure is applied and released. This normal reaction is called "pitting". Stage 2 is the spontaneously irreversible stage. The affected area is spongy to the touch, and the tissue does not indent when pressure is applied. Lymphedema is evident. The affected area swells and becomes fibrotic. Stage 3 is the lymphostatic elephantiasis stage. The swelling covers a large area, and damage is irreversible. The affected area is fibrotic.

Symptoms

Symptoms of lymphedema can cause exhaustion, uncomfortably swollen extremity, accumulation of fluid in the head and neck, skin discoloration, and deformity. Untreated lymphedema can cause serious infections, such as cellulites, lymphangitis, and lymphdenitis. This is because the fluid that accumulates in the tissue causes the channels in the tissue to enlarge and increase in number thereby reducing the amount of oxygen available to the body. This process hinders healing, and allows infection to set in. Severe cases may lead to skin ulcers. Left untreated for a prolonged period of time, lymphedema may lead to a cancer called lympangiosarcoma. Lymphedema can cause distortion of the affected body parts, and disfigurement. Along with the health problems, lymphedema can cause psychological discomfort.

Diagnosis

The diagnosis of lymphedema is difficult because the initial symptoms are subjective. Such symptoms may include a reported feeling of heaviness in the limbs, or a complaint that rings no longer fit. In the early stages, the edema of lymphedema may be so mild as to be extremely difficult to detect. More severe lymphedema may be diagnosed by measuring the difference in circumference between the affected limb, and normal limb. A difference of 4 centimeters may be used as an indication of the condition. The amount of fluid in the affected limb may be measured using bioimpedance. If it is suspected that lymphedema is present, the condition is monitored over time. Other diagnostic methods include lymphoscintigraphy (to trace the flow of fluid), MRI, CT, and duplex ultrasound (to monitor blood flow to rule out blood clot).

Grades of Severity

There are 5 grades of lymphedema based on symptom severity. Grade 1 involves mild edema. It affects the distal parts of the extremities. Swelling is mild, and the difference in circumference between the normal state and the affected state is less than 4 centimeters. Grade 2 involves moderate edema. The entire extremity or quadrant of the trunk is affected. Swelling results in a difference in circumference of less than 6 centimeters. Erysipelas may be evident. Grade 3a involves severe edema. The condition affects 1 entire limb, and truck quadrant. The difference in limb circumference is greater than 6 centimeters. Skin may show cornification, keratosis, or repeated episodes of erysipelas. Grade 3b involves massive edema. Two or more of the limbs are involved. Grade 4 involves gigantic edema. At this stage, the condition is also known as elephantiasis. Lymph circulation has been stopped almost completely. The head may be affected.

Surgical Treatment

Most physicians consider that surgery for lymphedema should only be attempted after conservative treatments have failed. Surgical treatment cannot cure lymphedema, but may improve the condition. Surgical treatment for lymphedema may take 1 of 2 approaches, excisional or physiological. Surgery might be recommended to remove excess tissue to make movement easier, or to increase circulation of the lymphatic fluid. Excisional techniques cut out affected tissue, and may involve skin grafting. Physiological techniques concentrate on improving drainage of the affected area. The lymphatic and venous systems are separate; surgery for lymphedema may involve bridging the 2 systems, encouraging the lymphatic fluid to drain through the venous system. The concern with surgery for lymphedema is the possibility of making the condition worse.

Sequential Pump Therapy and Complete Decongestive Therapy

There are 2 commonly used treatments for lymphedema. These are Sequential Gradient Pump Therapy, and Complete Decongestive Therapy (CDT). Sequential Gradient Pump Therapy uses a segmented pneumatic sleeve to squeeze out the excess lymphatic fluid. The sleeve fits over the affected area and is pumped full of air. The segments of the sleeve put pressure on the extremity in sequence, one after the other. This pushes the fluid along the affected area, and into circulation. Compression pumps may be used on the extremities and trunk. Complete Decongestive Therapy involves the use several modes of treatments including manual drainage, compression bandaging, exercise, and skin treatments. These treatments may be used in sequence. The pump may help break up fibrosis before the manual drainage part of CDT is started. Compression bandages aid the lymphatic system in reducing edema by adding resistance. Skin care helps prevent skin ulcers.

Olecranon Bursitis

The diagnosis of olecranon bursitis can be made from a physical examination, and report of symptoms. An x-ray may be taken to ensure that there is no joint damage. Acute olecranon bursitis may be treated by draining the excess fluid from the bursa with a needle. Medication may then be injected into the joint to reduce inflammation. Chronic olecranon bursitis is treatable, but the reason behind the continuing condition must be addressed. Individuals with the disorder must train themselves not to rest weight on their elbows. The elbows should be protected with elbow pads during sporting activities. Anti-inflammatory drugs may prove useful. Surgery may be necessary to drain or remove the damaged bursa. In case of infection, antibiotics may be indicated.

Bone Infection

The symptoms of bone infection include severe pain originating from the affected bone. Fevers, chills, nausea, and fatigue may be present. The skin overlying the infection site may be red, painful to the touch, and swollen. Osteomyelitis can worsen very quickly, and becomes more difficult to cure as it progresses. A history of recent injury may reveal the cause of the infection. A blood test will determine if the white blood cell count is elevated. An elevated while blood cell count is indicative of infection. An X-ray may determine if an infection is present, but a recent infection may not show up on x-ray. If a bone infection is suspected, a bone scan is indicated. A bone scan can provide a more detailed picture than an X-ray. An MRI can determine if an infection is present, and the stage of infection.

Osteomyelitis

Osteomyelitis is a bacterial infection of the bone. It can be chronic, or acute. Infection of the bone can occur in a number of ways. If another part of the body is infected, this infection can travel to the bone from the original infection site. This mode of infection is called hematogenous. Infection of bone most often occurs in this manner. An injury that includes an open wound may allow the entry of bacteria which may then travel and infect the bone. This most frequently happens when there is an open fracture. The disruption of the blood supply to a bone can also cause infection. This occurs most often in people with atherosclerosis, and diabetes. This type of bone infection most often occurs in the bones of the feet and toes.

Septic Arthritis

Septic arthritis is a joint infection. It generally spreads to the joint through blood circulation. An infected bone near the joint, or a penetrating wound, can also cause joint infection. The condition often occurs in individuals with an impaired resistance to infection. Individuals with diabetes, rheumatoid arthritis, leukemia, and autoimmune disease, for example, are at higher risk of developing septic arthritis. In individuals with normal resistance to infection, the bacterium involved is usually Staphylococcus aureus, or Gonococcus. In patients with impaired resistance, joint infection is often caused by Salmonella, and E coli. Although septic arthritis usually affects only 1 joint, multiple joints may be affected in individuals with poorly functioning immune systems.

Joint infection is indicated by pus in the synovial cavity. The cartilage is destroyed, and involved bone is broken down in a case of septic arthritis. Untreated, septic arthritis can cause fibrous, or bony, ankylosis. The diagnosis of this condition is based on joint pain that has no apparent cause paired with fever. Septic arthritis generally causes extreme heat in the joint itself, but some conditions, such as rheumatoid arthritis may hide this fact and complicate diagnosis. The heat may not be obvious if the infection is in the deep joints of the body. Severe pain is a symptom. Fluid aspiration from the affected joint and blood tests are used in diagnosis. Imaging studies such as x-ray, and MRI will show bone and cartilage changes. Bone edges may appear uneven. MRI may be particularly useful for the deep joints. Ultrasound is a useful tool in diagnosis to show effusion.

The success of treatment of septic arthritis depends upon the degree of damage done to the joint before treatment. Antibiotics must be administered at the earliest possible moment to lessen the degree of tissue damage. A delay in treatment may result in the destruction of the joint. Although early treatment with antibiotics is essential, antibiotics should not be started until the bacterium has been identified by culture of blood, synovial fluid, and affected tissue. The condition is extremely difficult to eradicate unless the appropriate antibiotics are administered. The use of inappropriate antibiotics before the bacterium has been identified will make it difficult later identify the bacterium causing the sepsis. Prolonged administration of antibiotics is advised. The condition tends to recur in individuals with a compromised immune system. Some cases may need lifelong treatment. The pus produce from the infection must be cleaned out of the joint. Passive movement is recommended.

Chondromalacia Patella

Chondromalacia patella is a tracking problem. It is a condition in which the patella does not travel in a straight line over the end of the femur. The action of the quadriceps muscle usually results in straight tracking, but in chondromalacia patella this is not the case. The patella gets pulled laterally, toward the outer femur. This causes the underside of the patella to rub against the bone of the femur causing inflammation and pain. The symptoms of this condition include mild pain in the area of the inner knee at rest, which is aggravated by activity, or standing after sitting for a significant length of time. The joint may feel tight, and mild swelling may be evident. The condition occurs more often in women than in men.

Clarkeâs Sign is an indication chondromalacia patella. In this test, the patient is asked to fully extend the leg, while the physician presses the patella down and distally. The physician asks the patient to contract the quadriceps gently. In a case of chondromalacia patella pain is felt with this action. Other tests include imaging studies such as x-ray, CT scans, and MRI. A CT scan provides the most information for this particular condition. Treatment starts with exercises to strengthen the quadriceps and Vastus medialis oblique, and to stretch the Achilles tendon. NSAIDS may be prescribed. A brace may be advised to support the patella. Surgical intervention involving arthroscopy may be recommended if surgical conservative fails. This involves debridement of the intra-articular surfaces. This may be combined with a lateral retinacular release. The tibial tubercle insertion of the patellar tendon can be elevated to rebalance the muscles acting on the patella.

Osteofibrous Dysplasia

Osteofibrous dysplasia is an aggressive, nonmalignant, fibrous tumor. The tumor affects adults and children, but it is usually diagnosed in children under the age of 10. In adults the site most commonly affected is the mandible. The mandible is only affected in adults with the disorder. In children, the tibia is most commonly affected. The tumor is also seen in other long bones, such as the fibula. The tumor appears to occur in males and females equally often. The cause of the tumor is unknown. The tumor is often asymptomatic, and presents as a painless mass. Osteofibrous dysplasia distorts and thins the bone cortex, and in the long bones, the tumor may cause bowing. The growth rate of the tumor is variable.

The tumor is often painless, but pain may be a symptom. Osteofibrous dysplasia presents with a localized swelling. If a long bone is involved, bowing anteriorly or anterolaterally is often present. Deformity of the bone may be present. The tumor may cause a fracture of the affected bone. In children, biopsy is generally not considered necessary for diagnosis and is avoided for fear of fracturing an already weakened bone. In adults, biopsy may be necessary to distinguish osteofibrous dysplasia from other conditions. Nonsurgical treatments are generally recommended until the bones are mature. This is due to the fact that the tumor tends to recur in immature bone, and surgical techniques may lead to fracturing of the weak bone. Pathological fractures are usually treated by casting. Bracing may help prevent pathological fractures of the legs. After skeletal maturity has been reached, the tumor can be resected, and necessary bone grafts performed.

Osteogenesis Imperfecta

Osteogenesis imperfecta is also known as brittle bone disease. Osteogenesis imperfecta is a genetic disorder of the bone. Individuals with this disorder are born with an inability to manufacture collagen, or an inability to manufacture normal, healthy collagen. This usually involves a deficiency in Type I collagen production, but this is not always the case. Individuals with this disorder may have less collagen than normal, or a poor quality of collagen. Collagen is an important component of bone, and it is needed to produce strong bones. Its absence causes weak and brittle bones which fracture easily. Osteogenesis imperfecta is an autosomal dominant disorder. The disorder can also occur as a result of a mutation. There are 4 generally recognized types of osteogenesis imperfecta. The types of osteogenesis imperfecta are categorized according to the level of collagen production, collagen quality, and severity of the disorder.

Type I and Type II

Type I osteogenesis imperfecta is the most common type, and the least severe type. In Type I osteogenesis imperfecta, normal collagen is produced, but in inadequate amounts. There is little bone deformity, but the bones fracture easily. The sclera (whites of the eye) may have a blue-gray cast. Type II osteogenesis imperfecta is a severe variation of the condition. It is generally lethal, causing death before one year of age. Infants with the disorder often die shortly after birth. The collagen produced by the body is of poor quality, and it is produced in inadequate amounts. Bones may break in utero. Death is generally due to respiratory problems, or bleeding in the brain (intracerebral hemorrhage).

Type III and Type IV

In Type III osteogenesis imperfecta, poor quality collagen is produced by the body, although adequate amounts are produced. Individuals with this condition are frequently short in height, and often exhibit severe bone deformities. The vertebral column may be curved. Fractures are often evident at birth. The whites of the eyes may be discolored. Symptoms may include brittle teeth, and respiratory problems. This type is progressive. Type IV osteogenesis imperfecta is a moderately severe type of the disorder. The collagen produced by the body is of poor quality but is produced in normal amounts. The bones are fragile, and fracture easily. Curvature of the vertebral column may be evident. Bone deformities are present, and they are mild to moderate in severity. Individuals with this disorder may be shorter in height than normal, and may have brittle teeth. The whites of the eyes are normal in appearance.

Treatment

There is no cure for osteogenesis imperfecta, and treatment centers on increasing the strength of the bone. The goals of treatment are to prevent fractures, and promote mobility. Physiotherapy helps to strengthen the muscles, and aids in maintaining mobility. Bisphosphonates are frequently prescribed to increase bone mass, which may reduce the incidence of fracture. Surgery may be indicated. Metal rods can be inserted in the intramedullary canals of long bones to increase their strength, and to prevent fractures. Scoliosis, which can be a symptom of osteogenesis imperfecta, may be corrected by spinal fusion. Surgery may be performed to relieve pressure on the spinal cord and brain stem in the case of neurological symptoms. Bone infections, which are associated with osteogenesis imperfecta, are treated with antibiotics as needed. Fractures are usually treated nonsurgically. Splinting and casting are kept to a minimum to prevent loss of bone strength.

Retrolisthesis

Retrolisthesis occurs when a vertebra slides back to overlap with the vertebra underneath. It is a result of degenerating discs, and occurs most often in the cervical and lumbar sections of the vertebral column. Radiographs show loss of space between the discs, and sclerosis of the vertebral body margins. Subluxation may show on radiograph. The condition may cause spinal cord compression resulting in pain and neurological abnormalities. Joint instability may be apparent. Treatment depends upon the severity and duration of the condition. Initial treatment involves medication to control pain, and a change in activity. Surgical treatment may be indicated in the case of neurological problems, or if pain continues despite conservative treatment. Although the degree of slip is not the deciding factor in treatment, an increasing deformity may indicate surgery as well.

Kyphosis

Kyphosis refers to an exaggerated forward curve to the spine. This results in a rounding of the back. A curve of more than 50 degrees is deemed to abnormal. There are several types of kyphosis including: postural kyphosis, Scheuermann's kyphosis, and congenital kyphosis. Postural kyphosis is the most common type of kyphosis. This is a flexible curve in the spine which often becomes evident during the teens. Radiograph reveals normal vertebrae and discs, and the condition is not painful. Postural kyphosis does not lead to problems in adulthood. Scheuermann's kyphosis also becomes evident in the teens. It involves a more extreme curve than that seen in postural kyphosis. The condition affects the thoracic, or lumbar, section of the vertebral column. Radiography reveals irregular and wedge-shaped vertebrae and discs. Congenital kyphosis results from the abnormal development of the vertebrae. The vertebrae may not form properly, or several vertebrae may be fused.

Kyphosis can be caused by many disorders. To give some examples, kyphosis can be the result of trauma to the spine, muscular dystrophy, infection, developmental disorders, and tumors. Cases of adult kyphosis may be the result of compression fractures caused by osteoporotic changes to the bone, or degenerative diseases of the vertebrae and disks, such as arthritis. Along with a rounded back, the symptoms of kyphosis may include back pain, stiffness in the spinal column, and fatigue. Difficulty breathing may be a symptom in severe cases of kyphosis. Neurological symptoms such as weakness in the legs, or paralysis may be complications of the disorder. Scheuermann's kyphosis resolves after the skeleton reaches maturity. Diagnosis is based on a physical examination, radiographs, radionuclide bone scan, MRI, and CT,

The treatment for kyphosis depends upon the type. There is no real treatment for postural kyphosis. It rarely causes pain, and exercise does little to straighten the back. This condition may improve over time on its own. Scheuermann's kyphosis may cause pain which is worsened by activity. The condition is often treated with exercises and anti-inflammatory drugs. A brace may be advised until the skeleton is mature. Congenital kyphosis may be progressive, and early surgical intervention is often indicated to help develop a more normal curve to the spine. Continued monitoring is necessary. Surgery may be recommended for a case of kyphosis if the curvature of the spine is greater than 80 degrees. The abnormal vertebrae may be straightened and fused. Kyphosis which is caused by infection or tumor may require surgery as well as treatment by medication of various kinds.

Scoliosis

Scoliosis is the curvature of the spine from side to side. In a case of scoliosis, the vertebral column looks like the letters "S" or "C". In this condition, some of the vertebra may be rotated. The disease can be congenital, idiopathic, or the result of another condition. Scoliosis has a hereditary component, but in most cases the cause of the condition is unknown. The disease can occur as a result of other disorders, but most often the condition occurs in healthy spines. The disease often originates in childhood, but can develop in adults. A case of scoliosis in adulthood may have begun in childhood, but gone undiagnosed. Other cases of adult scoliosis may be the result of degenerative conditions involving the vertebral column.

The symptoms of scoliosis include shoulders that aren't level, a listing posture, raised hips, and prominent shoulder blades. A physical examination for scoliosis includes Adam's Bend Test. In this test, the patient bends forward. If a hump on the back is present, scoliosis is suspected, and radiographs involving full length standing spine views are indicated. Although scoliosis does not usually cause problems in childhood, untreated scoliosis can result in continuing and severe back pain, deformity, and respiratory problems. Most curvatures of the spine require only monitoring, but if the curvature progresses, bracing of the spine is indicated. This can prevent the condition from becoming worse. A body cast may be advised. If the curvature is severe, or if an orthopedic brace does not prevent the worsening of the condition, surgery is indicated. Surgical techniques include spinal fusion, and internal fixation with rods and screws.

Lordosis

Lordosis is the excessive inward curvature of the spine. A certain inward curvature of the spine at the cervical, and lumbar, regions is normal. These curves serve to position the head over the pelvic region, and act as shock absorbers. When these curves become too pronounced, the condition is called lordosis. Lordosis is commonly called a swayback. Lordosis affects individuals if all ages. Although it is usually seen in the lumbar section of the vertebral column, it does occur in the cervical vertebrae. Lordosis in the lumbar region of the spinal column causes the buttocks to stick out excessively. Lordosis in the lumbar region can be painful, and can affect movement.

The curvature of the spine can be affected by certain diseases. These include the following: achondroplasia, which is a hereditary disorder of bone growth causing dwarfism; diskitis, which is an inflammation of the space between discs; kyphosis, which may cause a curve in the lower back to compensate for a curve higher in the back; obesity, which may cause lordosis by causing a backward leaning posture; osteoporosis, which may cause the vertebrae to weaken; and spondylolisthesis, which can cause the vertebrae to overlap. Lordosis can also be a benign juvenile condition. Lordosis does not always require medical intervention. If the curve is flexible, the condition is not generally of concern. If the curve is fixed, the condition should be evaluated medically.

Diskitis

Diskitis is the inflammation of the disk space between the vertebrae. This often occurs as a result of bacterial, or viral, infection. The infection does not originate in the vertebrae, or in the intervertebral space, but spreads from other sites through the bloodstream. It can also occur as a result of an auto-immune disorder. Diskitis usually co-occurs with vertebral osteomyelitis. The lumbar spine is the region most often affected by diskitis. The cervical spine and thoracic spine are the next most commonly affected regions. The disease usually effects children under the age of 10, but can also affect adults. The disease has a bimodal distribution, generally affecting children under ten, and adults over 50. Diskitis is an uncommon condition. It can occur after surgery, from urinary tract infection, and from soft tissue infections.

In children, diskitis may cause a low-grade fever, and pain and stiffness in the back. Abdominal pain may be present. The child may have trouble standing up, and may refuse to move. If forced to walk, the child may walk with an exaggerated curve to the spine. The disease is painful, and causes irritability. This condition can be confused with hip pain. Neurological deficits may be evident. Adult diskitis is more difficult to diagnose than the childhood condition. It has a slow course, may not be diagnosed until the disease is far advanced. Neck and back pain, along with localized tenderness, are the first symptoms. Movement causes the pain to worsen. The symptoms are not relieved by pain medication. Lower extremity weakness appears in severe cases. Fever, chills, and loss of weight may be present.

Radiography is useful in diagnosing diskitis, but symptoms may not be evident until several weeks after infection. The first symptoms to be seen on radiograph are narrowing of the disk space, irregularities of the endplates of the bone, and calcification around the affected area. As the disease progresses, the bone density increases. Subluxation of the vertebrae is evident. Nuclear medicine may be used in diagnosis. Ct scans are more useful than radiographs at showing early changes caused by diskitis. Using CT, hypodensity of the intervertebral disk, and the erosion of the endplate of the vertebrae can be detected. In addition, a CT can detect gases emitted by the bacteria at the infected site. MRI is the best technique for diagnosing diskitis. It can also distinguish between diskitis and other disorders, such as tuberculosis. Needle biopsy and surgical biopsy are also used in diagnosis.

Antibiotic treatment is tailored to the infective organism if at all possible. If this is not possible, broad-spectrum antibiotics should be administered. Antibiotics are given intravenously for 6-8 weeks. Persistent infection necessitates another biopsy, and continued administration of antibiotics. The patient should be immobilized in bed during early stages of treatment to allow affected vertebrae to fuse spontaneously in correct alignment. After the patient is allowed out of bed, the spine should be immobilized with a brace. A brace should be worn for 3-6 months. This may not prevent the collapse of the vertebrae, however. Pain medication is an important part of treatment. Surgery may be indicated if there is a neurological deficit, or spinal deformity involved. Surgery may also be necessary if the disease continues to progress. Surgery is performed to remove diseased tissues, take pressures off nerves, and ensure stability of the spine.

ACL Rupture

Rupture of the anterior cruciate ligament occurs frequently in people participating in fast moving sports that involve quick changes of direction. Examples of such sports are football, soccer, and basketball. An individual who has experienced an acute ACL tear will often report having heard a popping noise at the moment of injury. The individual may experience significant degree of pain at the time of injury. This is followed by a large amount of swelling in the injured knee. A notable decrease in range of motion may accompany the swelling. Instability occurring when rapid changes of direction are made is diagnostic. These symptoms indicate that a physical examination and imaging studies should be conducted.

Hallux Rigidus

Hallux rigidus is a form of degenerative arthritis that affects the joint of the big toe. The condition is progressive. It begins as hallux limitus, which is a condition where the mobility of the toe is limited. The condition progresses to the point where the joint becomes rigid, and cannot move. Hallux rigidus is a painful condition. Early symptoms include pain and stiffness of the joint during use, swelling, and inflammation. Later symptoms include pain during rest, pain wearing shoes, and pain in the hip, knee and lower back due to compensation. Hallux rigidus can be caused by trauma, inflammatory disease, faulty function, and abnormalities in the structure of the foot. The disease may also be hereditary.

The condition is generally diagnosed by means of patient report, symptoms, and x-rays. The patient may report difficulty and pain in walking, squatting, or bending. During examination, the toe will be manipulated to determine range of motion. Radiographs will be taken to determine the extent of the arthritic changes. Mild and moderate Hallux rigidus may be treated by changing shoe types. It is recommended that shoes with a large toe box and low heels be worn. Custom orthotics may help by changing the mechanics of walking. NSAIDS and injections of corticosteroids may reduce inflammation. Surgery may be required. Cheilectomy involves removing bone spurs, and part of the foot bone. If the joint cannot be preserved, it may be fused during an arthrodesis. The joint may be removed and replaced with an implant during an arthroplasty.

Piriformis Syndrome

Piriformis syndrome is a neuromuscular condition that causes deep pain in the buttocks. Symptoms of the syndrome include pain, a tingling sensation, and numbness along the path of the sciatic nerve. The piriformis tendon and the sciatic nerve are both found behind the hip joint. These paths of these 2 structures cross. The cause of piriformis syndrome is unknown. It has been suggested that this syndrome occurs when the piriformis tendon irritates the sciatic nerve. According to this theory, an abnormal tightness in the piriformis muscle and tendon causes pressure on the sciatic nerve, and reduces blood flow to this structure causing the syndrome in question. It has also been suggested that inactive gluteal muscles cause the condition. Another theory states that stiffness of the sacroiliac joints is responsible for the development of the disorder. The existence of piriformis syndrome is not universally accepted.

Piriformis syndrome is difficult to diagnose as the same symptoms occur with other disorders. Diagnosis is often a process of elimination. Disorders of the spine, sciatica, and tendonitis can all cause the same type of pain. Diagnosis may involve attempts to isolate the muscle to observe its functioning. There is no specific treatment for piriformis syndrome. Treatment involves rest, anti-inflammatory medication, physical therapy, and massage therapy. Recovery from this condition is difficult, and treatment is lengthy. The treatment of last resort for piriformis syndrome involves a surgical procedure in which the piriformis muscle tendon is released, or loosened. This is a large surgical procedure.

Advanced Cervical Stenosis

Cervical stenosis is the narrowing of the central canal of the cervical vertebrae. This condition can compress the spinal cord within the canal, and damage the long nerve tracts. Cervical stenosis can lead to loss of motor function. Symptoms include stumbling, and impairment in the functioning of the extremities. The first test conducted is the basic deep tendon reflex. Hyper-reflexivity is indicative of cervical stenosis. The second test checks for clonus. The examiner supports the ankle with one hand, and the patient's forefoot with the other. The examiner then forces the foot up into dorsiflexion. Clonus manifests in a rapid cycling of the foot between dorsiflexion and plantarflexion. A third test looks for Hoffman's reflex. This involves giving a downward flick to the middle finger. A subsequent downward movement of the index finger is indicative of cervical stenosis. Positive findings in any of these tests warrant further evaluation with MRI.

Pulmonary Embolism

A pulmonary embolism is a blockage of a lung artery by an embolus. This embolus may consist of fat cells, air, tumor cells, amniotic fluid, or clotted blood. A blood clot is the most common cause of pulmonary embolism. This is called a thromboembolism. This occurs when a blood clot from the circulatory system breaks loose, and enters the arterial blood supplying the lungs. Symptoms include respiratory difficulties, rapid respiration, and pain during respiration. A pulmonary embolism can lead to sudden death. Pulmonary embolism is an often fatal complication of fractures of the hip and pelvis. This disorder occurs with these types of fractures due to the interaction of trauma, immobilization, and swelling. These factors impair blood flow. Pulmonary embolism occurs much less frequently in cases of lower leg fracture. It is seen very rarely with upper body fractures.

Coxa Vara

Coxa varus is the outward turning of the hip. It is caused by a decrease of the neck-shaft angle of the femur. It can be congenital, acquired, or developmental. In Coxa vara, the neck-shaft angle of the femur is less than 125 degrees. This deformity can lead to partial, or complete, dislocation of the hip. The severity of Coxa vara is related to the length of the leg. More severe cases are those with an angle closer to 90 degrees. The more severe the case, the shorter the legs are. Like Coxa vara, 1 or both hips can be affected. If only 1 leg is affected, the legs will be of different lengths.

RICKETS

Rickets is a disease which affects adults and children. It involves the softening of the bones. This softening causes deformity and fractures. Although rickets is generally caused by a deficiency in vitamin D, a lack of calcium, or phosphorus, can also cause the disease. The presence of Vitamin D is necessary for the absorption of calcium, and phosphorus, which are necessary for healthy bones. Vitamin D may be ingested in the diet, or produced by the skin on exposure to the sun. There are certain risk factors for rickets. Children with dark skin, and children who are breast-fed and not exposed to the sun, are more likely to develop the disease. Breast milk is not high in Vitamin D. Rickets is a disease that usually affects children, although it can affect adults as well. A condition similar to rickets, called osteomalacia, occurs in adults. There is a rare genetic form of rickets called Vitamin D resistant rickets.

The symptoms of rickets involve the entire body. The symptoms affecting the skeletal system include bone pain, easily fractured bones, growth disturbances, and skeletal deformities. Skeletal deformities include such things as bowed legs, and arms, a misshapen skull, a projecting chest, and short stature. Other symptoms of rickets include muscle weakness, muscle spasms, hypocalcaemia, poorly formed teeth, and increased incidence of cavities. The deformities caused by rickets will persist into adulthood without treatment. The long-term consequences of rickets include bowed long-bones, and a curved spine. Without treatment during childhood, skeletal deformities may become permanent. Treatment in childhood can prevent many deformities from becoming permanent.

A number of methods may be used in a diagnosis of rickets. Blood tests may show low levels of calcium, and phosphorus. Serum alkaline phosphatase levels may be higher than normal. A test of arterial blood gases may show metabolic acidosis. Radiography may reveal a loss of calcium from the bones, or abnormalities in bone structure and shape. The tapping of the facial muscles may produce Chvostek's sign in an individual with rickets. Chvostek's sign is a spasm of the facial muscles. A bone biopsy will confirm rickets, but is rarely performed in diagnosis. Rickets is treated with supplements of calcium, phosphorus, or vitamin D. If the rickets is caused by a metabolic disorder, a special prescription for Vitamin D may be required. Bracing may be used to prevent deformities from developing, or to reduce existing deformities. Some types of skeletal deformity may require surgical correction.

TORTICOLLIS

Torticollis is commonly called wryneck. In this condition, the head is inclined toward 1 side while the chin is raised, and angled toward the opposite side. Torticollis has numerous causes, and it can be present at birth, or acquired. There are a number of congenital conditions that can cause torticollis, and it can also be acquired in childhood and adulthood. Whatever the cause of the torticollis, stress can cause symptoms to worsen. Chronic torticollis may cause physical and psychological disability. It may cause affected individuals to avoid social situations. The symptoms of torticollis are progressive, and change over time. This condition is included in a group of disorders involving abnormal positioning of the neck.

Some cases of congenital torticollis result from damage to the sternocleidomastoid muscle incurred from birth trauma, or malpositioning in the uterus. Other congenital cases are caused by cranial nerve IV palsy. Presentation depends upon the cause. In some cases of congenital torticollis, a soft-tissue mass develops in the affected sternocleidomastoid muscle. This development may take days, or weeks. With treatment, the mass usually disappears. Left untreated, the condition progresses. The mass eventually regresses, leaving a fibrous band of tissue. This causes the contracture of the neck. Torticollis resulting from palsy of the fourth cranial nerve is a neurological adaptation to nerve damage. It results from the attempt to maintain binocular vision.

Acquired torticollis can occur in children, or adults. Neck trauma can cause atlantoaxial rotatory subluxation. This condition causes the 2 vertebrae nearest the skull to slide against each other, resulting in tearing of the stabilizing ligaments. Infections of the ears and surgical removal of the adenoids can cause Grisel's syndrome. This is a subluxation of the joints in the cervical spine. It occurs because inflammation from infection causes the ligaments to become lax. Infections of the posterior pharynx can cause torticollis by irritating the nerves of the neck muscles. Torticollis can also occur when tumors at the base of the skull compress the nerves serving the neck. Some medications, such as antipsychotics and amphetamines, can cause torticollis. Idiopathic spasmodic torticollis occurs in people with a family history of the condition. This condition starts in individuals between the ages of 31 and 50. If left untreated, it becomes permanent.

The evaluation of a child with torticollis involves taking a detailed history. This helps determine if the condition is caused by birth trauma. The presence of torticollis is revealed by a decreased ability to bend and rotate to the unaffected side. In congenital torticollis, the right side is the affected side in 75% of cases. Radiographs should be taken to eliminate the possibility of bony abnormality in the cervical spine. MRI should be used if a structural problem is suspected. Vision problems should be ruled out by an eye examination. In all patients, cervical radiographs should be taken to look for bony trauma, or osteomyelitis. MRIs can rule out brain tumors, and herniated intervertebral disks. Trouble breathing, trouble swallowing, numbness in the arms and legs, incontinence, weakness in the extremities, and impaired speech indicate damage to the central nervous system.

Treatment of torticollis depends upon the cause of the disorder. Congenital torticollis caused by damage to the sternocleidomastoid muscle is treated with physical therapy and stretching. Surgery may be required in difficult cases. Torticollis caused by cranial nerve IV palsy should not be treated with physical therapy. In this case, treatment should focus on correcting the extraocular muscle imbalance. The treatment for acquired torticollis again depends upon the cause. Ligament damage is treated with traction, and bracing. Antibiotics and surgical debridement are used to treat infections of the posterior pharynx. Grisel's syndrome is treated with manipulation of the neck, or surgical resection. Tumors are treated surgically to relieve nerve compression. Spasmodic torticollis is treated with muscle relaxants, and anti-inflammatory drugs. Botulinum A toxin may be used to prevent muscle spasms.

Frozen Shoulder

Frozen shoulder is also called adhesive capsulitis. It causes pain, and loss of motion in the shoulder joint. The pain caused by the disorder is described as dull. Motion increases the pain. The use of the shoulder is impaired. It affects approximately 2% of the population. The disorder is most common among women 40-70 years of age. The cause of frozen shoulder is not well understood, but the condition follows a process. The capsule around the shoulder joint becomes thickened, and contracted. The condition has been described as having 3 stages. In Stage 1, the first symptom is a lessening of mobility. Pain level increases slowly. This stage lasts 6 weeks to 9 months. In Stage 2, the pain starts to decrease, but mobility does not improve. This situation may last for 4 to 9 months. In Stage 3, mobility slowly improves over a period of 5 to 26 months.

Frozen shoulder is diagnosed based on physical examination, patient history and self-report of symptoms. Frozen shoulder develops sometimes as a result of being held immobile due to an injury. Certain factors increase the risk of developing frozen shoulder. These include hypothyroidism, hyperthyroidism, diabetes, bursitis, Parkinson's disease, osteoarthritis, and heart disease. Imaging studies are sometimes conducted to eliminate other possible causes of the symptoms. Although frozen shoulder usually resolves on its own, this may take several years. Treatment generally involves controlling pain, and increasing range of motion. Anti-inflammatory medications are prescribed for pain and inflammation. Physical therapy includes range of motion exercises and stretching exercises. Nerve blocks may be used to treat that does not respond well to NSAIDS.

Surgical intervention may be required if all other treatments have failed. Before surgery, it must be considered that most cases of frozen shoulder will resolve with time. The goal of surgical intervention is to release the contracted joint capsule. Manipulation of the shoulder under anesthesia, and arthroscopy are often used to this end. Manipulation of the joint involves forcing the shoulder to move. This causes stretching, or tearing of the capsule. Arthroscopy involves cutting through the contracted portions of the capsule. These 2 techniques are often used together. Surgery for frozen shoulder is usually successful. Physical therapy after surgery is essential to maintain mobility. Recovery may take 6 weeks to 3 months.

Plantar Fasciitis

Plantar fasciitis is the inflammation of the plantar fascia. This fascia extends from the part of the foot near the toes to the heel. The pain involved with plantar fasciitis is generally felt where the fascia attaches to the heel bone. Plantar fasciitis is a painful condition caused by stress to the underside of the foot. The pain is most extreme on first weight bearing in the morning, and decreases after a few steps. The condition is associated with long periods of weight bearing activity. Individuals who are obese, and those who spend a long time on their feet, are more likely to experience this condition. The wearing of shoes with little arch support may contribute to the condition.

Treatment for plantar fasciitis is effective, although it generally takes 6 to 18 months for the condition to heal. Treatment includes stretching the Achilles tendon and plantar fascia, rest, taping, and arch support. NASAIDS may be used to relieve pain and inflammation. Supportive foot wear can help ease the condition. Injections of corticosteroids may relieve discomfort on a permanent or temporary basis. These injections may be painful, however. For this reason, a local anesthetic is often used before the corticosteroid injection. Night splints worn to keep the foot flexed dorsally may help decrease morning foot pain. Surgical intervention may be used as a last resort. This may involves a plantar fascia release, but this technique may cause other problems. A fasciotomy is an effective surgical treatment. This involves inserting a needle into the plantar fascia, and moving it back and forth to break up the fibrous tissue that has formed.

Gout

Gout is a kind of arthritis. It results from an excess of uric acid in the body. Uric acid is a waste product that is normally excreted in urine by the kidneys. In gout, either too much uric acid is produced, or it is not excreted properly. The uric acid in the body is deposited as crystals in various parts of the body. The crystals are sharp, and cause pain and swelling. Although the uric acid is usually deposited in joints, it can also be deposited under the skin, in the soft tissues, and in the kidneys, or urinary tract. Affected joint often appear red, and swollen. The disease affects the big toe most often, but the other joints in the extremities can also be affected. Men are much more likely than women to develop gout. Gout has 4 stages. These are as follows: asymptomatic, acute, intercritical, and chronic.

The symptoms of gout appears suddenly, and often during the night. Individuals with gout are often awakened during the night by extreme pain in the big toe, or foot, or ankle joint. The sensation has been described as a stretching or tearing pain. The skin over the affected area is hot, red, and swollen. The pain may be so bad that the weight of a blanket is unbearable. The wearing of shoes may be impossible. The base of the big toe is the joint most frequently affected, but most other joints can be affected. The first attack of gout generally subsides within 10 days. Gout has a very strong tendency to recur. Subsequent attacks occur more frequently, are longer lasting, and involve numerous joints. Gout may lead to persistent inflammation, and become chronic.

Gout can be caused by a number of factors. There seems to be a hereditary component, as many people with the disease have a relative with the disease. Some medications, such as drugs to treat high blood pressure, can cause gout by interfering with the excretion of uric acid in the urine. This interference causes an accumulation of uric acid crystals in the body. Some kinds of food can trigger gout. These foods include seafood, and liver. Beverages such as coffee and tea can contribute to the development of gout. Alcohol can trigger attacks. Physical events such as strokes, heart attacks, surgery, and trauma can cause the development of the disease.

Gout may be suspected from symptoms, and the patient's description of the pain. There are laboratory tests to aid in the diagnosis of gout. Blood tests may reveal a high level of uric acid, but this is not necessarily diagnostic. Many people have high levels of uric acid in the blood and never develop gout. The level of uric acid in the urine can also be tested. A high level suggests gout. A needle may also be inserted into the painful joint to withdraw fluid from the joint. This fluid is put under a microscope and examined for the presence of uric acid crystals. It is important to find the cause of the disease.

There is no cure for gout, but it can be controlled. The goal of treatment of this disease is to relieve the symptoms of current attacks, prevent future attacks, and prevent damage to the joints. The cause of the disease must be established. Medication is used to treat acute attacks and chronic gout. Nonsteroidal anti-inflammatory drugs are commonly used to treat gout. NSAIDS reduce the pain caused by the disease, reduce swelling, and decrease stiffness in the joints. These drugs do not prevent damage to the joints, however. There are many kinds of NSAIDS, and different NSAIDS work better for different people. Corticosteroid injections can reduce swelling and inflammation in an affected joint. Colchicine is also used to reduce inflammation, but this drug may cause gastrointestinal problems after a short time of use. Diet may have to be altered to treat acute gout, and prevent future attacks.

WHIPLASH

Whiplash is a named used to describe neck sprains caused by the neck being thrown forcefully forwards and/or backwards. The action of the whiplash causes tearing of the fibers of the muscles of the neck. This tearing results in pain, and lessened mobility. This type of injury is often sustained in car accidents when the car is struck from behind. It can also result from other types of accident. Approximately 20 percent of individuals in cars struck from the rear develop pain in the neck region. A small percentage of these individuals develop chronic problems leading to chronic pain, and disability. Symptoms of whiplash include neck stiffness, neck pain, headaches, low back pain, and dizziness. More severe symptoms include ringing in the ears, blurred vision, impaired memory and concentration, and sleep problems.

Most whiplash injuries involve soft tissues such as the disks of the spine, muscles, and ligaments. A diagnosis of whiplash is often a diagnosis of exclusion. These injuries cannot be seen on standard radiographs. Specialized tests may be needed to assess a suspected whiplash. These tests may include CT scans, or MRI. Digital motion x-rays which allow the ligaments to be examined in motion, can aid in diagnosis. Whiplash injuries used to be treated by immobilization with a cervical collar, but this has fallen out of favor. Currently, the belief is that early movement is desirable. The cervical collar may be used intermittently rather than continually. The application of ice for the first 24 hours will prevent swelling. After 24 hours, gentle exercise should be started. No single treatment is used, but medication, exercise, physical therapy, traction, and massage have proved useful. Continuing symptoms may require surgical intervention.

Lateral Patellar Malalignment

Lateral patellar malalignment causes pain with knee flexion and extension. Such malalignment is generally the result of a muscle imbalance. The initial treatment of this problem is conservative, and involves bracing and physiotherapy to strengthen the quadriceps muscle. If these methods fail to relieve the pain, surgical intervention may be indicated. The surgical technique used to treat lateral patellar malalignment is a lateral release. Lateral tension on the patella is decreased by cutting the tissue to the lateral patellar retinaculum by means of arthroscopic surgery. This release allows the patella to slide back into its central position. To prevent a recurrence of the condition, the patient must continue with strengthening exercises to maintain the positioning of the patella.

Carpal Tunnel Syndrome

In carpal tunnel syndrome the median nerve becomes compressed as it travels through the carpal tunnel. The condition can be congenital, but repetitive motion can also cause this condition. Repetitive motion can cause inflammation of the structures within the carpal tunnel, and the transverse ligament, and lead to compression of the median nerve. Carpal tunnel syndrome causes pain in the thenar eminence of the hand which radiates into the thumb, index finger, long finger, and ring finger. Decreased sensation in this area may be experienced. Loss of strength in the hand will result from prolonged compression of the nerve. Symptoms are usually worse in the morning, and prolonged activity aggravates the condition.

Phalen's test was developed to test for carpal tunnel syndrome. The patient is asked to press the backs of the hands together with a wrist flexion as close to 90 degrees as possible. This position is to be held for at least a minute. Numbness resulting from this test is indicative of carpal tunnel syndrome. The speed at which the numbness occurs in this test indicates the severity of the condition. The more severe the condition, the faster the numbness occurs. Tinels' sign is a test to detect nerve irritation. In this test, the patient's wrist is tapped along the portion of the median nerve that runs through the carpal tunnel. A tingling sensation, like pins and needles, is indicative of carpal tunnel syndrome. If these tests are positive, EMG testing can be conducted to confirm diagnosis.

Tennis Elbow

Tennis elbow, or lateral epicondylitis, involves inflammation at the lateral elbow. In this condition, the tendinous insertions of the wrist extensor muscles become inflamed due to overuse. The history of the injury should include the patient's occupation, hobbies, and information regarding hand dominance. The pain will usually be localized to the lateral epicondyle of the elbow, but it may spread into the forearm. On examination, range of motion should be tested, and the injured elbow palpated to determine areas of tenderness. As further confirmation of the diagnosis of lateral epicondylitis, the patient should be asked to extend the wrist, and hold this position while a flexion force is applied to the hand. This flexion force will pull directly on the inflamed tendons and cause pain. A thorough neurovascular assessment of the arm and hand should be conducted.

Assessment of Extensor Tendon Function in Thumb and Fingers

Tendon ruptures, or tendon lacerations involving the thumb and fingers are easily missed injuries. As these can cause serious disabilities if left untreated, all patients with a suspected injury to the upper extremity should undergo evaluation for tendon function. To determine if the functioning of the thumb extensor tendons is impaired the patient is asked to raise the thumb straight up in a "thumbs up" gesture. Inability to do this indicates a problem. To test the functioning of the remainder of the finger extensors, the patient is asked to stick all of the fingers straight out. If the extensors are functioning properly all of the fingers will be straight. The strength of each finger should be tested, as weakness may be a sign of partial rupture. Any deficit should be reported to the orthopedic surgeon.

Assessment of Flexor Tendon Function in the Thumb and Fingers

The flexor tendons should be examined if there is an injury to the upper extremity. The flexors of the thumb can be tested by asking the patient to flex the tip of the phalanx while the proximal phalanx is held steady. Ability to do this indicates a competent tendon. The functioning of the two flexor tendons in each finger must be evaluated by testing each finger one at a time. To test the functioning of the deep tendon the patient is asked to flex the tip of the finger at the distal interphalangeal joint while the middle phalanx is stabilized. To test the functioning of the superficial flexor tendon the patient asked to flex the digit at the proximal interphalangeal joint while the proximal phalanx is stabilized. Any deficit found on this examination should be immediately addressed by the orthopedic surgeon.

Iliotibial Band Syndrome

Iliotibial band syndrome is also called iliotibial band friction syndrome. This condition is called ITBS, or ITBFS for short. This condition causes lateral knee pain, and is commonly caused by running, cycling, hiking, and weight lifting. The iliotibial band is a superficial strip of thickened tissue located on the outside of the thigh. Its starting point is on the outside of the pelvis, and it runs over the hip and knee. During the action of running, the band moves from the back of the femur to the front. The insertion point of the band is just below the knee joint. The iliotibial band stabilizes the knee joint. Activity causes the iliotibial band to rub over the lateral femoral epicondyle. This rubbing, combined with continued extension and flexion, may result in inflammation, or irritation.

There is a range of symptoms associated with iliotibial band syndrome. Symptoms can occur anywhere along the length of the band. Symptoms may include a stinging sensation felt on the outside of the knee, or along the length of the iliotibial band, swelling of the band where it crosses from the front to the back of the femur, and pain below the knee. The pain associated with the disorder may worsen with activity. Pain may persist after the activity has been stopped. Iliotibial syndrome can also occur where the band attaches to the hip. Pain at this site is not likely due to a sports injury, but occurs often with pregnancy as the connective tissues in the area loosen. Iliotibial band syndrome in the hip is also common in the elderly.

Iliotibial band syndrome often presents with pain on palpation of the lateral knee. Pain increases when the patient is standing with the knee flexed to an angle of 30 degrees. Physical examination involves the use of Ober's test. This test is used to determine the tightness of the iliotibial band. The patient is asked to lie on the table on the unaffected side of the body. The unaffected hip and knee are flexed to 90 degrees. The examiner aligns the affected leg with the rest of the patient's body by abducting and extending the leg. The affected leg is then adducted. If the iliotibial band is of normal length, the leg will adduct without pain. If the iliotibial band is abnormally short, adduction will be difficult and cause pain to the lateral knee. Tightness prevents the smooth functioning of the iliotibial band contributing to the development of iliotibial band syndrome.

Iliotibial band syndrome can be prevented by building strength in the muscles of the hips. Exercises to stretch the iliotibial band and gluteal muscles can aid in preventing the development of this condition. Runners with iliotibial band syndrome are advised to reduce running distance for a period of time, and to run only on flat ground. After the cessation of pain, distance can be increased gradually. Persistent pain requires complete rest from running for about 2 weeks. If pain still persists, rest for another month is advised. As the injury improves, activity can be resumed slowly and gradually. Changing the running route may help prevent recurrence of symptoms as running the same route constantly may put more stress on one side of the body. Rest, cold compresses, and elevation should be used to treat acute symptoms. NSAIDS will relieve inflammation and pain. Corticosteroid injections may be prescribed.

Surgery is rarely used to treat iliotibial band syndrome. It is only used in cases where the condition persists after 6 – 12 months of conservative treatment. It should be a treatment of last resort, and only used when all other treatments have failed to produce relief. Patients who refuse to change their exercise routine are generally the population treated by surgery. Surgery is only performed after arthroscopic examination has ruled out other possible causes for the pain. Surgical treatment involves an iliotibial band release-excision performed using arthroscopic techniques. Rehabilitation includes stretching, gradual introduction of exercise, deep-tissue massage non-steroidal anti-inflammatory drugs (NSAIDS), and strengthening exercises for the quadriceps femoris, and gluteus medius muscles.

Shoulder Impingement

Shoulder impingement is a common cause of shoulder pain in adults. It is caused by the shoulder blade exerting pressure on the rotator cuff as the arm is raised. In shoulder impingement, the acromion of the shoulder blade pushes on the muscles of the rotator cuff causing pain, and hindering the motion of the shoulder. The pressure created by the shoulder blade may cause bursitis, or tendonitis. A tear of the rotator cuff may also be present. This condition is commonly seen in athletes engaged in sports requiring overhead motion. The motions involved in tennis, baseball, and swimming may cause the shoulder impingement. Certain jobs may also increase the risk of developing shoulder impingement. Paper hanging, construction, and painting may increase risk for the condition. The condition may also occur for no apparent reason.

The symptoms of shoulder impingement may be mild at first, and become increasingly severe. A low level discomfort may be present continuously. Pain may radiate from the front of the shoulder down the arm. Reaching movements, or lifting, may cause sudden pain. Shoulder impingement can cause localized swelling and tenderness. As the condition progresses, the condition may cause pain at night. It may result in the loss of strength, and affect range of motion. Pain may be experienced on lifting, or lowering the arm. Activities requiring the arms to be used behind the back may cause extreme pain. In severe cases, the condition may result in a frozen shoulder. The area of injury may be tender to the touch.

An examination for shoulder impingement includes a physical examination to determine areas of pain, and to determine the range of motion possible. Radiographs and other imaging studies will determine if there are any bony abnormalities. For example, an outlet view radiograph may show a bone spur on the leading edge of the acromion which is sometimes the cause of the condition. An MRI can be used to examine the area for signs if inflammation, or fluid, in the bursa and rotator cuff. MRI can identify any torn sections of the rotator cuff. An impingement test which involves the injection of a regional anesthetic can be used to confirm the diagnosis of shoulder impingement.

Conservative treatment for shoulder impingement is tried first. Rest and the avoidance of overhead movements that cause pain are recommended at this stage. Nonsteroidal anti-inflammatory drugs may be prescribed for pain. Stretching exercises may be recommended to improve range of motion in the shoulder. A cortisone injection may relieve pain, and help restore range of motion. Conservative treatment may take several weeks to months to have an effect. Surgical treatment may be advised if conservative methods fail to resolve the problem. The goal of this surgery is to increase the space available for the rotator cuff. Surgery may be arthroscopic, or use open techniques. Possible surgical procedures include subacromial decompression, and anterior acromionplasty. In most cases of surgery, the anterior edge of the acromion is removed to create more space. Other shoulder conditions may be repaired at the same time.

Rehabilitation following surgery may involve the use of a sling. This will take weight off of the affected area, relieve pain, and allow healing. When the pain starts to subside, the sling can be removed. Although the sling should be removed as soon as possible to get the shoulder moving, it should not be removed too soon; the healing tissue must be protected. Exercises will help restore the range of motion of the shoulder, and the strength in the arm and shoulder. Therapy will start with passive motion. The rehabilitation program will be individualized based on needs and surgical findings. It may take 2 to 4 months for complete recovery, and for the pain to subside completely.

Medial Epicondylitis

Medial epicondylitis is a condition known by many names. It is also called flexor origin syndrome, reverse tennis elbow, and golfer's elbow. This condition is a tendonitis affecting the flexor wad at the anterior medial epicondyle of the humerus. It is the most frequent cause of pain in the medial elbow, although it occurs less frequently than lateral epicondylitis. Medical epicondylitis affects twice as many men as women. It occurs most often in individuals between 20 – 49 years of age, but can occur in all age groups. Certain sporting activities, like golf, baseball, and tennis raise the risk of developing medial epidondylitis. Repetitive work can also cause the condition. Although medial epicondylitis is most often caused by overuse, it frequently begins as a result of an acute injury.

The main symptom of medial epicondylitis is pain over the medial epicondyle. This pain gets worse with flexion and pronation of the wrist. The ulnar nerve may be involved as evidence by a tingling or numbness that spreads into the ring, and little fingers. This tingling or numbness may be intermittent, or constant. Soreness to the touch over the anterior part of the medial epicondyle is the most commonly reported symptom. The condition does not usually affect range of motion of the elbow or wrist. Symptoms of neuropathy of the ulnar nerve are often evident. These symptoms may include decreased sensation in the areas served by the ulnar nerve. Severe cases may be associated with weakness, and muscle atrophy.

An individual with medial epicondylitis feels pain with resisted wrist flexion, and perhaps with resisted elbow flexion. In an examination for medial epicondylitis, radiographs are generally taken of the elbow to determine if there are any associated problems, such as osteoarthritis, avulsions, or loose bone fragments. Anteroposterior and lateral views are usually sufficient to diagnose this condition, but if loose bodies are suspected, oblique views of the joint are advised. Loose bodies may be suspected due to a clicking sensation in the elbow joint, or if the joint appears to be catching. Valgus stress radiographs are indicated if medial instability appears to be a possibility. An MRI is not usually considered necessary for the diagnosis of this condition. A nerve conduction study and electromyography are advised if the ulnar nerve is involved.

Occupational and physical therapy are recommended treatments for medial epicondylitis. Rest, icing of the injury, compression, and bracing are used to reduce inflammation and decrease pain. Rest is generally recommended for 1-6 weeks. The use of ice is particularly important with acute injuries. The area over the ulnar nerve should not be iced, however. Compression of the elbow by means of a medial counterforce brace, with a pad placed over the flexor pronator wad is the usual treatment for this condition. A wrist splint may be worn keep the wrist in a neutral position to allow it to rest. If the ulnar nerve is also involved, a nighttime elbow extension splint may be advised. This splint allows 30–45 degrees of flexion, and protects the nerve from further damage. After the injury has become less painful, exercises are recommended to strengthen the flexor-pronator muscles. Ultrasound treatments may be recommended.

If conservative methods fail to relieve symptoms, medial epicondylitis may be treated with a regional anesthetic, and steroid injections. Care must be taken to avoid injecting into the tendon, or nerve. The number of injections should be limited to 3 to reduce the chance of tendon atrophy, or rupture. Although cortisone injections provide short-term relief, this treatment is not a permanent cure. Surgical intervention for medial epicondylitis is rarely necessary, but may be indicated if other methods fail. Surgical techniques to treat this condition include epicondylar debridement, the surgical decompression of the ulnar nerve, and release of the flexor origin. Surgical treatment has been found to be effective in over 80 percent of surgical cases.

Intersection Syndrome

Intersection syndrome is also called crossover syndrome. The condition is caused by repeated actions of the wrist. The condition affects the forearm and wrist, and pain is usually experienced a few inches above the wrist. At this site, 2 muscles that join to the thumb run over top of 2 wrist tendons. The muscles involved in this condition control the movement of the thumb. Their actions pull the thumb out and back. These muscles are called the extensor pollicis brevis, and the abductor pollicis longus. The tendons involved in this condition are attached to the extensor carpi radialis brevis muscle, and the extensor carpi radialis longus muscle. These 2 wrist tendons extend the wrist. The tendons of the wrist are covered with tenosynovium which allows the tendons to glide easily over the surrounding tissues. If the extensor tendons are overused, the tenosynovial covering becomes inflamed, and swollen.

Intersection syndrome is a painful condition. The swelling of the tenosynovium prevents the wrist tendons from gliding smoothly. This friction between the wrist tendons and other tissues causes a squeaking noise, and results in a creaking sensation. This phenomenon is called crepitus. Pain begins at the intersection point of the tendons and muscles involved in the condition. This is about 3 inches up from the wrist. The pain may radiate down the wrist to the thumb, or along the forearm. Swelling and redness may be apparent at the intersection of the tendons and muscles. Movement is painful. No special tests are required to diagnose intersection syndrome, and it is diagnosed in the physician's office.

Nonsurgical treatment of intersection syndrome involves stopping, or decreasing, the activities that are aggravating the tendons. Frequent breaks when performing repetitive hand and thumb movements are essential in healing the condition. Hand movements that irritate the nerves should be avoided all together as much as possible. The wrist should be kept in a neutral position. A special splint may be needed to help with this. A thumb-spica splint keeps the wrist and thumb joints still, and quiet. Resting the joints allows healing of the tendons. Anti-inflammatory drugs can reduce inflammation of the tenosynovium, and relieve pain. The use of ice can also accomplish these ends. If these treatments don't ease the symptoms, cortisone injections may help. The effects of the cortisone are not permanent, however. In very rare and severe conditions, surgery may be recommended. This involves cutting away some of the thickened synovium. This is called a tendon release.

If nonsurgical treatment is to be successful, results will be seen in 4–6 weeks although symptoms may not disappear completely during this time. Continued use of the thumb splint may be necessary to control symptoms. Activities that caused the problem should be curbed to avoid a return of symptoms. If surgical intervention was necessary, symptoms start to abate immediately. Pain in the area of the incision may continue for several months. For the first while, the hand should be kept elevated above the heart. The fingers and thumb should be moved gently. The stitches should be kept dry. Stitches are removed 10-14 days after surgery. Physical therapy sessions should be attended for 6 to 8 weeks, and full recovery will require several months.

Avascular Necrosis

Avascular necrosis is also called osteonecrosis, aseptic necrosis, and ischemic bone necrosis. It is a disease that results from the loss of blood supply to the bone. The loss need not be permanent to cause avascular necrosis. The bone dies without a constant blood supply, and collapses. If the loss of blood supply occurs near a joint, the joint surface often collapses. Avascular necrosis can affect any bone in the body, but most often affects the shoulder, knee and hip joints. The ends of long-bones are most frequently affected. Avascular necrosis has many causes, including, but not limited to, steroid use, trauma, decompression sickness (Caisson disease), thrombosis, and vasculitis. In some cases of avascular necrosis, no cause can be found. These cases are called idiopathic. The disease usually strikes individuals between the ages of 30 and 50.

Bone normally breaks down and is repaired. In avascular necrosis, however, the bone cannot repair itself as fast as it breaks down. Left untreated, the disease leads to bone collapse, and pain. Arthritis develops when joints collapse. The amount of disability resulting from avascular necrosis depends upon the area involved, and the amount of damage. Avascular necrosis is usually diagnosed by means bone scintigraphy and MRI. Both these methods can detect bone changes early in the disease. Standard radiographs may not be sensitive enough to detect changes early in the disease, but will show changes in later stages of the disease. Radiographs may be used to monitor the course of the disease. A Ct may be useful in determining the extent of damage to the bone.

Conservative treatment for early avascular necrosis may involve reduced weight bearing, and NSAIDS. Surgery is usually eventually required. Core decompression involves the surgical removal of the inner layer of bone allowing the formation of more blood vessels. An osteotomy reshapes the bone, and reduces stress on the damaged area. A bone graft can help support the joint. Grafting of arteries and veins can add to the blood supply. Avascular necrosis often affects the hip. The most common treatment is a total hip replacement. A less drastic form of hip replacement is metal on metal resurfacing. This involves the removal of only the head of the femur instead of the whole neck. The free vascular fibular graft is another method of treating avascular necrosis of the hip. In this method, part of the fibula and its blood supply, is transplanted to the head of the femur.

Wrist Drop

Wrist drop is a symptom with many causes. In this condition, the wrist and fingers cannot be extended, and hang loose when the arm is held out, palm down. Wrist drop may occur when the extensor muscles and their tendons, or the radial nerve supplying the extensor muscles are not working properly. It is most often caused by damage to the radial nerve. Wrist drop can be caused by lead poisoning, as lead poisoning can damage the radial nerve. Repetitive motion can cause wrist drop by damaging the radial nerve. Prolonged pressure on the radial nerve, perhaps caused by the use of crutches, or by habitual leaning on the elbow, can cause wrist drop by damaging the radial nerve. Neuromuscular disease can also cause wrist drop. The condition is found in individuals of all ages.

As wrist drop has many causes, patient report of symptoms and a medical history can help in diagnosis. The assessment for wrist drop involves nerve conduction velocity studies to determine if the radial nerve is the source of the problem. X-rays can be used to rule out the presence of bone spurs and fractures which may be pressing on the radial nerve. MRI may be used to distinguish between possible causes of the problem. Treatment depends upon the cause of the condition. Initial treatment may involve splinting of the wrist, and occupational, or physical therapy. Surgical intervention to remove bone spurs may be required to remove pressure from the radial nerve. Other causes of pressure on the radial nerve may also need surgical intervention. Neuromuscular disorders require medication.

Physical Examination for Suspected Fracture

In examination for a suspected fracture, any unnecessary pain, or discomfort, to the patient must be avoided. First, the history of the injury must be obtained. Next, the affected area should be visually examined for signs of damage, such as deformity, swelling, or skin breakdown. A neurovascular examination is in order as damage to blood vessels, or nerve tissue is a serious complication. Particular attention should be paid to the area distal to the fracture. The lack of a pulse in this area, or a lack of sensation, is a serious finding, and the orthopedic surgeon should be informed. The areas distal and proximal to the injury should be palpated with particular attention paid to nearby joints. A thorough examination can ensure additional fractures aren't overlooked. A physical examination can help determine what imaging studies should to be completed, and ultimately what treatment options should be considered.

MRI

Magnetic resonance imaging (MRI) allows accurate diagnostic visualization of the internal structures of the body. It can produce multiple cross-sectional images. MRI uses radiofrequency waves and a magnetic field to produce its images. MRI is best used in the examination of soft tissue structures, but can also be used to visualize bony structures. This technique is highly accurate in detecting abnormalities and injuries. MRI does not use radiation to produce images, and this can alleviate concern about extensive testing. There are drawbacks MRI. MRI studies can take up to an hour to complete which becomes a problem for patients who are claustrophobic. Another consideration is the magnet which is a part of the scanner. Patients with certain metallic implants, such as pacemakers and vascular filters, cannot have MRI because the magnetic field can be strong enough to disturb the functioning of these implants, or to displace them.

CT

CT (computed tomography) uses radiation to produce cross-sectional images. CT is capable of producing a series of images. The CT scan is a rapid exam which makes it much more tolerable than MRI for some patients. The radiation used in CT, however, is a concern for some patients. Ionizing radiation is potentially cancer causing. Although the risk incurred with 1 scan is small, it increases with additional studies. CT produces better images of bones and fractures than MRI is capable of producing. Soft tissue may not show up as clearly as desired in a CT scan, however. To counteract this phenomenon, an injected contrast can allow better visualization. Some patients may react to the contrast with allergic symptoms. Patients with certain types of implants may not be able to have MRI, and may be referred for a CT scan instead.

Physical Therapy Treatments

Ultrasound is a passive mode of treatment. The high frequency sound waves generated by the ultrasound equipment travel deep into the tissue and warm the soft tissues. This treatment promotes healing and relaxation. Heat is beneficial to the healing process as it increases circulation, promotes relaxation, and decreases pain, and stiffness. Ice is used to decrease pain. It does this by slowing the rate at which the nerve pulses travel. Ice also prevents, and decreases inflammation. Physical exercise uses exercises which are designed to stretch the muscles, and relieve pain and stiffness. Electrical muscle stimulation uses electrical impulses to contract muscles. This aids in preventing muscle atrophy, and stopping muscle spasms.

Bone Growth Stimulators for Fracture Healing

A bone growth stimulator is an appliance that delivers a low level electrical current to a fracture site. This device is thought to increase metabolic activity in the injured area resulting in faster healing, and more robust bone formation. Research suggests that the bone growth stimulator can have positive effects on acute and slow healing fractures. Certain bones are more likely to heal poorly, perhaps resulting in nonunion. Poor healing can be due to fracture location, fracture shape, and blood supply. For this reason, bone growth stimulators are often used on acute fractures of the scaphoid, fifth metatarsal base, and tibia. Different types of stimulator are worn for different lengths of time. Proper education ensures best results from a particular device. The stimulator must be fitted to the patient's injury in a way which places the highest concentration of electrical current as close to the fracture as possible.

Evaluation of Stability of Collateral Ligament of Elbow

To begin, the elbow is inspected for swelling, cuts, or deformities. The patient is asked to flex, extend, supinate, and pronate the joint. These movements are repeated while the joint is palpated to determine if it is intact. To test the collateral ligaments, the examiner grasps the patient's upper arm with the left hand so that the hand covers the joint line. With the right hand, the examiner firmly holds the forearm and applies varus stress to the joint. As the stress is applied, the left hand is used to feel for a space at the lateral joint line. No slackness will be felt if the lateral collateral ligament is undamaged. To test the medial collateral ligament the procedure is repeated, but a valgus stress applied. The examiner should feel for a space, or slackness, over the medial joint line. The affected elbow should be compared to the unaffected elbow.

Examination of Collateral Ligaments of Metacarpal-Phalangeal Joints

The metacarpal-phalangeal (MP) joints are easily injured by a twisting force on the hands. The collateral ligaments of the MP joint are still somewhat slack when the fingers are completely extended. These ligaments become tight when the MP joint is flexed to 90 degrees. This action increases the stability of the joint. This fact needs to be understood in an examination of the joint. The joint is first inspected for swelling, areas of redness, or deformity. The joint is palpitated to locate areas of tenderness. The stability of the MP joint is tested by evaluating the tautness of the ligaments. The metacarpal is held with one hand and the proximal phalanx with the other hand. The finger is then flexed to 90 degrees, and the proximal phalanx is wiggled side to side. No laxity should be felt on either side of the joint. Any slackness could indicate damage.

Brief Neurovascular Exam of Hand

Visually inspect the hand for deformity, and skin damage. Examine the coloring of the skin, and the distribution of hair, as vascular abnormalities can affect these. Palpate the hand for tender spots. Check the radial and ulnar arterial pulses. Check each digit for capillary refill. To check the median nerve sensory function, lightly touch the palmar tip of the index finger. To examine the motor function of the median nerve, ask the patient to abduct the thumb. To test the sensory function of the ulnar nerve, palpate the pad of the little finger. To test the motor function of the ulnar nerve, ask the patient to abduct and adduct each finger. Test the sensory function of the radial nerve by palpating the dorsal web area between the thumb and first finger. Check the motor function of the radial nerve by asking the patient to extend the thumb.

Key Components of Initial Interview of Orthopedic Patient

The first step is to discover the nature of the orthopedic problem. Determine if it is acute or chronic in nature. Ask about the source, and nature of the problem. Determine the type of pain the patient is experiencing (e.g. sharp or dull, constant or intermittent). Have the patient rate the severity of the pain/symptoms. A common scale is 1-10 with 1 being very minor pain, and 10 being severe pain. Question the patient regarding the location of the pain. Inquire if the pain stays localized, or if it radiates to another part of the body. Ask the patient what activities make this pain worse, and which ones alleviate the symptoms. Have the patient outline all previous treatments that have been received for this problem. Inquire about the patient's overall health, co-existing medical conditions, and previous surgical history.

X-Ray Evaluation of Long Bone Injury

Several points must be kept in mind regarding radiographic studies of long bone injuries. One of the most important issues is the number of views needed to evaluate the severity of the fracture. The x-ray is a 2 dimensional representation of a 3 dimensional injury. This necessitates anterior-posterior, lateral, and oblique views to fully evaluate the fracture. A bone can seem to be in alignment on one view even if there is gross displacement obvious from a different angle. All available radiographs should be used in evaluation of the fracture. Radiographs should be taken of the joint above and below the injured bone to check for possible additional fractures or dislocations.

Important Terms

Medial - The medial line is the midline of the body. The term medial refers to being nearer to the midline of the body. The eye is medial to the ear. The knee has medial and lateral sides.

Lateral - Lateral is essentially the opposite of medial in that it refers to being further away from the midline of the body. For example, the ear is lateral to the eye.

Proximal - Proximal is a descriptive term that refers to being closer to the center of the body. The knee is proximal to the ankle.

Distal - Distal is a descriptive term that refers to being further from the center of the body. For example, the ankle is distal to the knee.

Abduction - Abduction is the movement of a body part away from the midline.

Adduction - Adduction is the movement of a body part toward the midline.

Circumduction - Circumduction is the movement of a body part in a circular motion.

Rotation - Rotation is the movement of a part of the body around a central axis.

Dorsiflexion - Dorsiflexion involves the bending of the foot from the ankle joint upward.

Plantar flexion - Plantar Flexion involves the bending of the foot downward from the ankle joint.

Eversion - Eversion involves the turning of the foot so that the sole of the foot in inclined outward.

Inversion - Inversion involves the turning of the foot so that the sole is inclined inward.

Flexion - Flexion involves the bending of a joint.

Extension - Extension involves the straightening of a joint.

Pronation - Pronation involves the turning of palm downward, or the eversion and abduction of the foot.

Supination - Supination involves the turning of the palm upward, or the inversion and adduction of the foot.

Appendicular skeleton - The appendicular skeleton consists of the arms and legs. It contains 126 bones.

Axial skeleton - The axial skeleton consists of the cranium, vertebral column, sternum, and ribs. There are 80 bones in the axial skeleton.

Condyle - A condyle is a rounded process at the end of a bone which serves as a surface of articulation with another bone.

Crest - A crest is a long elevated ridge on a bone.

Epicondyle - An epicondyle is a process on a bone. Epicondyles are located above a condyle, and are sites of attachment for ligaments and tendons.

Foramen - A foramen is a natural opening in a bone through which anatomical structures such as nerves, ligaments, and blood vessels pass. The foramen magnum, for example, is a large hole in the occipital bone which provides passage for the spinal cord.

Fossa - A fossa is a depression on a bone.

Diaphysis - The diaphysis is the shaft of a bone.

Physis - The physis is also known as the epiphyseal plate, or growth plate. It is located between the epiphysis and metaphysis. It is the site of longitudinal bone growth.

Epiphysis - The epiphysis is the end of a bone.

Metaphysis - The metaphysis is located between the diaphysis and epiphysis. Active bone formation occurs at this site.

Periosteum - The periosteum is a thin dense fibrous tissue which covers the bones. The periosteum is 2-layered. The inner layer is important for bone growth and reshaping. The outer layer protects the bone. The periosteum contains blood vessels, and nerves.

Endosteum - The endosteum is a thin layer of connective tissue which lines the inner part of bones that have a medullary cavity.

Fovea - A fovea is the name for a cup-shaped depression on a bone. A fovea is smaller than a fossa.

Head - The head of a bone is the proximal end.

Process - A process is a natural projection from a bone.

Trochanter - A trochanter is a large process on the femur serving for the attachment of muscle. There are two trochanters. The greater trochanter is situated on the outer and upper part of the shaft of the femur. The lesser trochanter is located at the junction between the shaft and neck of the femur.

Tuberosity - A tuberosity is a nodule on a bone which allows for the attachment of muscles and ligaments. It is larger than a tubercle.

Bursa - Bursae are sacs containing synovial fluid which serve to reduce friction, and act as cushions between structures that move against each other. They are found between muscles, or in places where tendons pass over bone. Tendon sheaths are bursae which wrap around tendons.

Synovium - The synovium is the soft thin membrane lining the inside of a joint cavity. The membrane produces and absorbs synovial fluid, which lubricates the joint and nourishes the cartilage.

Fascia - Fascia (plural fascae) is a band, or sheet of connective tissue that covers structures, such as muscles, blood vessels, and nerves and isolates them.

Meniscus - A meniscus is a disk of cartilage that cushions a joint, and protects the bones from the effects of friction.

Delayed union - Delayed union refers to a lengthened healing time. This could result from a pathology, mechanical problem, or trauma.

Nonunion - A nonunion refers to any fracture that fails to heal in a reasonable time frame. Any number of circumstances can lead to a nonunion. Poor positioning, or improper immobilization, of a fracture can cause nonunions. There are instances when certain fractures, such as those of the scaphoid, fail to heal under the best circumstances.

Malunion - A malunion is a situation in which a fracture heals in any anatomically incorrect position. Certain fractures, such as the fifth metacarpal, will allow for some malunion without altering function. Some fractures, the distal radius for example, need nearly perfect anatomical reduction to restore normal function. If a patient presents with a fracture that has gone on to a malunion, and it is causing problems, a corrective osteotomy may be performed.

Osteomyelitis - Osteomyelitis is an acute or chronic inflammation and infection of the bone and bone marrow. The infection can be bacterial, or fungal in nature. The infection may start in another part of the body, and travel to the bone through the bloodstream.

Osteonecrosis - Osteonecrosis refers to the death of bone tissue. There are several forms of osteonecrosis. It may be post-traumatic, non-traumatic, or idiopathic. It often results from a disease, or trauma which destroys the blood supply to the area in question.

Osteoma - Osteoma is a bone tumor.

Osteoporosis - Osteoporosis is a loss of bone density resulting from a loss of calcium. The disorder results in weak bones which break easily. Osteoporosis affects more women than men. In women, bone density decreases significantly after menopause.

Osteopenia - Osteopenia is a loss of bone mass to an abnormally low level. Osteoporosis and osteomalacia are types of osteopenia.

Ankylosis - Ankylosis is an abnormal stiffness in a joint caused by injury or disease. It is often the result of rheumatoid arthritis.

Anthralgia - Anthralgia refers to pain in a joint.

Osteochondritis - Osteochondritis refers to the inflammation of bone and cartilage.

Osteogenesis imperfecta - Osteogenesis imperfecta is a genetic, congenital condition which results in the production of defective type I collagen by the body. The condition is characterized by deformed, brittle, and easily fractured bones.

Osteogenesis - Osteogenesis refers to the formation of bone.

Osteomalacia - Osteomalacia is a condition involving an abnormal softening of the bone due to a loss of bone mineral. The condition results from inadequate amounts of calcium and phosphorus in the blood which in turn results from a deficiency of vitamin D.

Osteoarthritis - Osteoarthritis is a disease of aging. It is a degenerative joint disease in which the articular cartilage wears away causing bone to rub on bone. The ensuing friction between the bones causes pain.

Arthrotomy - Arthrotomy is the process of surgically opening a joint by an incision. An arthrotomy can be done as a therapeutic measure, or as part of a larger procedure. For example, in a total knee arthroplasty, an arthrotomy is made to give the surgeon access to the joint surfaces to be replaced.

Osteotomy - Osteotomy refers to the cutting of bone. As with an arthrotomy, an osteotomy can be done as a treatment measure. It may be used, for example, to correct a fracture that has healed with an incorrect angle. An osteotomy may also be part of a larger procedure. An example of this is a greater trochanteric osteotomy, performed to allow lateral access to the hip joint.

Osteoclasis - Osteoclasis is the intentional fracturing of a bone in order to correct an abnormality in structure.

Arthroscopy - Arthroscopy is the process of inserting a small camera into a joint to allow visualization. This is often done through a small incision to minimize soft tissue disruption. Arthroscopy can be done as a diagnostic tool, or can be utilized in the treatment of a specific condition, such a knee meniscus repair.

Arthroplasty - Arthroplasty is the replacement of a joint. This is frequently done using an artificial implant. A hip replacement, for example, involves the use of a femoral implant with a corresponding acetabular cup. In some instances, an artificial implant is not employed, but a repositioned tissue is used to reconstruct the joint. For example, in arthroplasty of the thumb carpal-metacarpal joint, the joint is repaired using the palmaris longus tendon.

Arthrotomy - The term arthrotomy means an incision into a joint.

Desmotomy - The term desmotomy means an incision of a ligament.

Myotomy - The term myotomy means an incision of the muscle.

Neurotomy - The term neurotomy means an incision of a nerve.

Osteotomy - The term osteotomy means the cutting of a bone.

Tenotomy - The term tenotomy means an incision of a tendon.

Arthrectomy - The term arthrectomy means the excision of a joint.

Ostectomy - The term ostectomy means the excision of a bone.

Sequestrectomy - The term sequestrectomy means the excision of a dead bone.

Arthrodesis - The term arthrodesis refers to the removal of the cartilage of a joint performed to encourage the bones to fuse.

Synostosis - A synostosis refers to the fusion of bones which are normally separate. This fusion could be surgical, or natural.

Arthrodesis - Arthrodesis is the surgical fusion of a joint. This procedure is performed for the purpose of pain relief, and to increase stability of the joint. It is performed mostly on wrists and ankles.

Arthrocentesis - Arthrocentesis involves the removal of synovial fluid from a joint by needle puncture. This procedure is conducted for the purpose of diagnosis, or to remove excess fluid.

Laminectomy - Laminectomy refers to the surgical removal of the lamina of the vertebra to relieve pressure on a nerve root. The lamina is the posterior arch of the vertebra.

Synovectomy - Synovectomy is the surgical removal of the synovial membrane found within a joint. This procedure is conducted when the membrane is inflamed or damaged. It is a treatment for rheumatoid arthritis.

Disarticulation - Disarticulation of a joint refers to the amputation through the joint.

Dislocation - A dislocation occurs when a joint alignment is disrupted due to the displacement of a bone from its usual position. This injury can constitute a true medical emergency due to possible injury to nearby nerves, or blood vessels. A dislocation should be reduced (put back into place) as soon as possible.

Subluxation - A subluxation is essentially a partial dislocation. A joint will exhibit a shift in its usual alignment, but the bones that make up the joint will maintain some contact. These injuries will sometimes reduce spontaneously.

Fracture - A fracture is a crack, or break through a bone. This can range from the mild bending of a bone to an open fracture in which the broken bone ends have pierced the skin.

Angulation - Angulation is the deviation of the broken bones from the normal position.

Rotation - Rotation is the turning of a bone fragment on the central axis.

Allograft - An allograft, also referred to as allogenic graft and homograft, is the transplant of cells, tissues, or entire organs from an organism of one species to another organism of the same species.

Autograft - An autograft, also referred to as autologous graft and autochthonous graft, is the transplant of cells, tissues, or entire organs from one part of an organism's body, to another site within that same organism.

Xenograft - A xenograft, also called a heterograft, heterologous graft, and heteroplastic graft, is the transplant of cells, tissues, or entire organs from an organism of one species into an organism of another species.

Isograft - An isograft, also called a syngraft, is the transplant of cells, tissues, or entire organs from one organism to a genetically identical recipient.

Chondroporosis - Chondroporosis is the process by which spaces appear in cartilage. This process occurs normally, and in abnormal conditions. Ossification is a normal process which involves chondroporosis.

Chondrolysis - Chondrolysis is a process involving the loss of articular cartilage. It results from the breakdown of the cartilage matrix and cells.

Chondroplasia - Chondroplasia is a process in which chondrocytes, which are specialized cells, form cartilage.

Chondropathy - Chondropathy is a term referring to disease of cartilage.

Chondrotomy - Chondrotomy is a term referring to the surgical cutting of a cartilage.

Chondroplasty - Chondroplasty is a term referring to the surgical repair of a cartilage.

Chondroosteodystrophy - Chondroosteodystrophy is a group of disorders of the cartilage and bone.

Closed reduction - A closed reduction is the repositioning of a fracture without use of an incision. The fracture is stabilized by external methods.

Open reduction - An open reduction is a method of repositioning a fracture which makes use of an incision at the fracture site.

External fixation - External fixation involves the use of pins, or screws inserted through the skin, and the bone. These are positioned above and below the site of the fracture. These pins, or screws, are then attached to a metal bar, or bars, placed against the injury outside the skin. This creates a frame, which is removed after sufficient healing has taken place.

Internal fixation - Internal fixation involves surgery. The bones are realigned and then held in place with screws, metal plates, or rods through the marrow space.

Dehiscence - Dehiscence is the separation of the edges of a wound. This is sometimes a complication of surgery that occurs as a result of poor wound healing. Risk factors for dehiscence include diabetes, obesity, and advanced age.

Cauterization - Cauterization is the use of heat to stop bleeding. The 2 types of cauterization in general use in medicine today are electrocautery, and chemical cautery.

Anastomosis - Anastomosis is the joining together of 2 structures. It usually refers to a connection created between 2 hollow structures, such as blood vessels, or sections of intestine.

Debridement - Debridement refers to the removal of dead, damaged, contaminated, or infected tissue. This process is carried out to improve healing. Debridement may be by surgical, mechanical, chemical, or autolysis means. Further, maggots can be used to debride in cases where the tissue is necrotic.

Adhesion - An adhesion is the joining together of normally separated tissues. It can be caused by inflammation of the tissues, injury to the tissues, or surgery. Adhesions can result in painful conditions, or conditions that interfere with normal functioning. An adhesion can be treated by surgery, but there is a possibility that this will make the condition worse.

Plica - A plica is a fold, ridge, or pleat, in the synovial tissue of the joint capsule. It often results from injury, but can be a developmental condition. Plica is generally diagnosed, and treated, through arthroscopic procedures.

Atrophy - The term atrophy refers to the wasting away of a body part. This condition can be caused by poor nutrition, poor circulation, inadequate nerve supply to the area, decrease in hormone levels, lack of use, and disease.

Bifurcation - A bifurcation is the splitting of an anatomical structure into 2 parts.

Casting, Splinting, and Orthopaedic Appliances

Cast Application

Casts are made of plaster, or fiberglass. The type of fracture, or injury, needs to be identified to determine the type of cast needed. Before the cast bandages are applied, a stockinette is placed on the affected area to protect the skin. The stockinette should be long enough to extend past both ends of the cast so that it may be folded back to hold in the cast padding. The stockinette must lay flat against the skin, with folds kept to a minimum, to help reduce friction. Next, cast padding, also called Webril, is rolled onto the injured area. This padding protects the skin and bony protuberances. The entire area to be casted must be well padded, but extra padding should be placed over bony prominences. The padding is rolled on with each roll overlapping the previous roll by 50%. Next, the wet cast bandages are rolled on. Plaster casts are made from rolls of dry muslin that have been coated with calcium sulfate. The cast is now molded to fit the area being casted. When the plaster bandages are wet, a chemical reaction occurs between the water, and calcium sulfate, causing heat to be produced, and the cast to harden. Warm water increases the heat given off by the plaster. The temperature of the water used in the application of the cast affects its setting time. When cold water is used, the cast takes longer to set. Although it starts to feel hard 10 - 15 minutes, plaster casts usually set completely in 24-48 hours. Pressure should be applied to keep the fracture in place until the cast dries.

Synthetic Fiberglass Casting Tape vs. Plaster of Paris Casting Tape

Although fiberglass casting tape is more expensive than plaster tape it has definite advantages. The material is lighter, and more comfortable. This can be beneficial particularly if a cast is going to be required for an extended period of time. Fiberglass casts are more durable than plaster casts, and are less likely to need repair, or replacement. Fiberglass casts are more radiolucent than plaster casts. This reduces the need for casts to be removed for the purpose of taking x-rays of the fracture. It should be noted that although fiberglass casts are more water resistant than plaster casts the padding still gets wet and retains moisture. It is still advised therefore, that fiberglass casts be kept dry as possible.

General Cast Care Instructions for Patients

The patient should be advised to keep the new cast away from body and clothing until it is dry to avoid transferring the cast material. The patient should be told not to stick any foreign object into the cast as this could result in damage to the skin and possibly start an infection. Many individuals with casts use long objects to scratch inside the cast. This should be discouraged. The visible padding of the cast should not "picked at" as this could result in the rough edges of the casting material irritating the skin. The patient should be instructed not to get the cast wet. When bathing, or showering, the cast should be kept out of the water, or covered with a waterproof barrier. Finally, the patient should be told to contact the doctor if there is any problem with the cast, or if numbness should develop, or pain increase.

Cast Removal

Begin by describing the process to the patient, as the noise and vibration can be disturbing. Mark on the cast the places where it will be cut. Try to avoid cutting over any bony prominences. Making cuts on opposite sides of the cast will make removal easier and faster. Apply only enough pressure with the cast saw to push the blade through the cast material. Once the blade is through, retract it, and move the saw down the cut line. Don't just drag the blade down the cast. Retracting the blade will allow for more control, and minimize the risk of inflicting saw burns. When the cast has been cut fully on both sides, separate the 2 halves with the spreader tool. Bandage scissors are used at this point to cut the padding under the cast to fully remove device.

Short Arm Cast

A short arm cast is typically applied for stable wrist fractures. The top of the cast should start on the forearm about 2 inches under antecubital crease to prevent the cast from irritating the upper arm. The bottom of the cast should end proximal to the metacarpal heads. The padding should therefore end at the distal palmar crease. This arrangement will allow the patient to flex the metacarpal-phalangeal joints, preventing stiffness. The area over the ulnar tuberosity should be well padded, as this prominence could be subject to discomfort and skin breakdown due to friction. The thumb should be well padded, and the casting tape should be placed in such as way as to allow free movement of the digit. An injury to the thumb may require a thumb spica addition.

Long Arm Cast

A long arm cast extends at least to the mid-biceps region of the upper arm. The elbow joint is usually casted to be at a 90 degree angle. The forearm is in a neutral position. Conservative treatment calls for unstable wrist fractures to be treated with a long arm cast. Such a cast helps to prevent wrist flexion and extension, and eliminates radial-ulnar supination and pronation. For these reason, a long arm cast is also the best choice for fractures involving both bones of the forearm. A long arm cast also ensures stability for patients who may not abide by activity restrictions. A short arm cast may slide off the arm of a younger patient whose forearm muscles have not developed sufficiently to support the cast. A long arm cast solves this problem.

Thumb Spica Cast

This cast is used to treat stable, reduced fractures, injuries to the ligaments of the thumb, and non-displaced scaphoid fractures. The stockinette is applied first as for a short arm cast. A length of 1 inch stockinette is then unrolled to cover the thumb. The cast padding is rolled to cover the thumb. The short arm cast is applied using 2 inch casting tape. When the thumb is reached, the casting tape is wrapped around the thumb and then around the hand. On the second pass, the casting tape is brought from the other side so that the second loop "locks" the thumb in place. Cutting the casting tape partially may allow for a better fit around the thumb. Excess stockinette at the ends of the cast and at the tip of the thumb is folded over. Different injury patterns determine whether or not the thumb interphalangeal joint should be immobilized.

Munster Cast

A Munster cast limits the supination and pronation of the arm without completely preventing flexion and extension of the elbow. The cast is applied in a standard fashion, in the manner of a long arm cast. During application however, the cast is extended to just above the distal biceps. Once it has hardened, the proximal portion of the cast is trimmed around the elbow joint. The closer to the distal humerus/olecranon the cast is cut, the more movement of the elbow will be allowed. Patient compliance with medical recommendations is essential, because of the amount of movement the cast allows. Although movement will help prevent stiffness in the elbow joint, the importance of immobilization should not be disregarded. This is also called a supracondylar cast.

Short Leg Cast

Short leg casts are used typically for fractures of the foot and ankle. The proximal end of a short leg cast must stop below the tibial tubercle to prevent damage, or irritation, to the tibial tubercle and the patellar tendon. This also prevents the cast from injuring the soft tissues at the posterior knee while it is flexed. The short leg cast must be constructed so that the distal end covers the plantar surface of the foot and extends to the metatarsal heads. The toes must be exposed. Generally, the ankle joint should be casted at 90º to prevent unnecessary tightening of the Achilles tendon. The medial and lateral malleoli must be padded in order to prevent skin damage. Care should be taken to prevent damage to the area over the anterior ankle joint, and the heel. Additional layers of casting tape applied around the heel helps prevent cast breakdown.

Long Leg Cast

The long leg cast is often used in the treatment of non-displaced fractures of the lower leg and knee. The cast extends from the upper thigh to the metatarsal heads. The cast is molded with the knee in 15-20 degrees of flexion. This degree of flexion serves 2 important purposes. The flexion prevents the lower leg from rotating in relation to the femur. This is particularly important in the treatment of tibia fractures which have a spiral component to them. Another function of this degree of knee flexion is that it permits ambulation with crutches as the leg can swing freely. This keeps the patient from becoming bedridden which can lead to co-morbid conditions.

Long Leg Cylinder Cast

The long leg cylinder cast is a useful auxiliary treatment in injuries to the anterior knee. Patellar fracture, rupture of the quadriceps tendons, and rupture of the patellar tendons can all cause impairment in the extensor mechanism of the knee. Healing often requires a long period of keeping the knee extended. This is best obtained through casting. The leg is casted from mid thigh to the Achilles tendon in a position of full extension. The distal end of the cast should be particularly well padded to protect the Achilles tendon from pressure, irritation, and friction. To prevent the cast from slipping, extra cast padding should be added at the proximal end. The casting tape should be rolled as usual, and molded to the area above the knee to stop the cast from sliding down the leg.

Uni-Valving and Bi-Valving a Cast

Post-injury swelling in an extremity could cause ischemia if the limb is encased in a cast. Ischemia necessitates the removal of the cast. If the cast is causing discomfort, but not compromising neurovascular health, the cast could be split. Bi-valving is a method which involves cutting the cast as for removal, and slightly separating the edges with a cast splitter. Uni-valving involves making a single cut in the cast. These techniques will decrease the pressure inside the cast, but still allow the cast to support and immobilize the affected limb. A neurovascular examination should be conducted after valving to determine if enough pressure has been relieved. If there is any uncertainty, the cast should be completely removed. Valving will allow the patient's swelling to completely subside before a new cast is applied. Valving can also be used if surgery is going to be performed in the near future.

Serial Casting

Serial casting is used to correct joint position, and improve mobility. The cast is changed at specific intervals, to slowly induce a change in the joint position. This technique can be used to treat a deformity caused by an imbalance of the muscles. A child suffering from cerebral palsy might benefit from this technique. Serial casting can also be used in the treatment of an acquired injury, such as a rupture of the Achilles tendon. An Achilles tendon rupture treated with serial casting involves initially casting the foot in extreme plantar flexion. When a certain amount of healing has occurred, the cast is removed and a new cast decreasing the amount of plantar flexion is applied. This cast will remain in place for a period of 7-10 days. This process is repeated until a normal range of motion has been re-established.

Delbert, Dehne, and Gauntlet Casts

A Delbert cast is a short leg cast that prevents lateral movement while allowing dorsiflexion, and plantar flexion. It is applied, and then trimmed away from the anterior and posterior ankle, and the heel.

A Dehne cast is also called a three-finger spica cast. Used to treat fractures of the navicular, it is comprised of a section covering the thumb, and a separate section enclosing the index, and middle fingers.

A gauntlet cast is used to treat fractures, or dislocations, of the metacarpals and phalanges. It is a short cast that extends from above the wrist to cover part of the palm of the hand. It often has an extension to control 1 or more of the digits.

Cast Shoes

The terms cast shoe, bunion shoe, and post-op shoe describe the same device. It is a removable appliance with a rigid bottom that prevents the foot from flexing during walking, and weight bearing. The cast shoe is frequently worn over a cast to allow walking without damage to the cast. The shoe also has a treaded bottom to prevent slipping. Certain types of foot fractures which do not need rigid fixation, but benefit from some support, can be treated by use of a shoe cast. Non-displaced fractures of the fifth metatarsal's proximal tip fall into this category. A cast shoe may decrease the pain caused by toe fractures during the acute phase of the injury.

Hip Spica Cast

A hip spica cast is used to prevent movement of the hip joints, and/or thighs to allow healing after injury. The cast is often used in the treatment of fractures of the femur, or damaged hip joints. The length of the cast varies with the injury, but generally extends from the middle of the chest to an area below the knees. If both hips or both thighs are affected the cast will cover both knees. If only one side is affected only 1 knee will be covered. A space is left in the cast to allow the wearer to use the bathroom. The cast is usually used in the treatment of injuries in children. The cast is usually applied under general anesthetic. The iliac spines, ribs, and back must be well padded to protect these bony sites.

Windowing a Cast for Wound Observation

The cast window allows for the monitoring of underlying wounds on casted extremities. Prior to applying a cast, a diagram is made of the affected extremity indicating the location of the wound. The cast is applied, and allowed to dry. Referencing the diagram created, the area of the wound is outlined. A wide margin is included so that the surrounding tissue can be observed. A saw is used to cut along the borders of the window and a cast splitter used to raise the window from the body of the cast. The cast padding and stockinette under the cast tape is removed carefully to avoid tissue damage. A margin of padding is left to help protect the skin. The wound should be fully exposed. Padding is reapplied over the windowed area, and the cast shell is placed back on top. This is held in place with an ace wrap.

Splinting vs. Casting

Splinting is often the treatment of choice for musculoskeletal injuries. Splinting allows for swelling at the injury site which is important in situations of acute fracture and sprain. A splint is easily removed, which allows easy access for continuing observation of the injury. This is particularly important in surgical cases as it allows the wound to be examined to make sure it is healing properly. A splint can be used as a transitional treatment after casting before normal activities are resumed. A splint can be removed for the purpose of exercising the injured area, or for physical therapy. A splint can be removed for normal activities, but replaced to protect the injured area while sleeping, or replaced as needed for support.

Wrist, or Hand, Dorsal Blocking Splint

A dorsal blocking splint is used on the dorsal side of the wrist, or hand, for the purpose of limiting extension. This splint is particularly useful in the treatment of patients who have had a surgical repair of the flexor tendons of the wrist or fingers as it will prevent passive and active extension, thereby preventing stress to the site of repair. Fractures of the volar plate of the fingers can often be treated non-operatively with blocking splints. Blocking splints keep the affected finger in flexion and hold the bony fragments together. The dorsal blocking splint must not be too tight or too loose. The splint must fit firmly to provide necessary support, but not too tightly or it may create problems.

Conservative Treatment Options for Clavicle Fractures

The majority of clavicle fractures are treated conservatively. Clavicle fracture treatment is designed to relieve pain, and immobilize the fracture. Complete immobilization of clavicle fractures is not necessary for proper healing. The two main methods of treatment are slings and figure 8 splints. Slings decrease pain by taking the weight of the arm off of the clavicle. The second treatment option is the figure 8 splint. This type of splint has a padded harness which comes across the front of each shoulder and travels around to the back. The straps in the back have clips that allow tightening of the splint. This apparatus helps to hold the shoulders back in order to keep the fractured ends of the clavicle together for better healing. The splint must be kept tight to work, and it is considered uncomfortable to wear.

Splinting a Mallet Finger

A mallet finger is caused by damage to the extensor mechanism of the distal interphalangeal (DIP) joint of a finger. It can be a soft tissue injury, or a bony injury. A soft tissue mallet finger involves a rupture of the extensor tendon. A bony injury involves an avulsion fracture of the distal phalanx. These injuries are largely treatable with conservative measures such as an extension/hyperextension splint. Although the splint can be made of a number of materials, alumifoam splints are superior because they are pliant. The proximal interphalangeal joint may be left unsplinted to allow the range of motion. The splint must not be removed prematurely, as the newly formed fibrous connections can be disrupted if sufficient healing hasn't taken place. This takes 6 – 8 weeks. Premature use of the joint can result in a chronic extensor lag.

Volar Wrist Splint

A volar wrist splint is used to provide temporary support for acute wrist injuries, and to immobilize the wrist after surgery. The first step in applying the splint is to pad the wrist and hand with Webril. The length of splint required to cover the area from the proximal forearm to the metacarpal heads is measured against the patient's arm. The plaster, or fiberglass, tape is rolled to the desired length with a thickness of ten to twelve layers. After the casting tape is rolled out, eight to ten thicknesses of cast padding are rolled out. The casting tape is then wet in a bucket of water, drained, and positioned on top of the padding material. The splint is placed so that it starts just below the metacarpal heads and extends proximally along the volar forearm. The splint is held in place while an ace wrap is applied.

Hinged Elbow Brace

A hinged elbow brace supports the elbow medially and laterally, but still allows flexion and extension of the joint. The brace prevents stress from inward and outward movement, which is helpful when treating injuries to the collateral ligaments of the elbow. The hinged elbow brace is used in transition from elbow immobilization to full range of motion activities. The elastic sleeve of the brace must be fitted snugly to the patient's upper arm and forearm, without cutting off the circulation. The brace may have straps to adjust the tension above and below the elbow. The medial and lateral hinges must be placed perfectly, or flexion and extension may be hampered. The brace material may cause irritation to the patient's skin. To help prevent this, a length of casting stockinette may be worn under the brace. This will help prevent irritation, and prevent perspiration from dirtying the brace.

Upper Extremity Posterior Splint

Posterior splints of the arm are used to stabilize fractures, immobilize the elbow joint after surgery, and in the treatment of acute elbow injuries. The splint extends distally from the posterior surface of the upper arm to the wrist or hand. The actual ending of the splint will depend on its purpose. The degree of flexion at the elbow will depend upon the injury, but normal placement to stabilize the injury is 90 degrees. The ulnar nerve and bony prominences of the elbow must be accommodated when applying padding. Multiple layers of padding around the elbow should be applied, with special attention to the olecranon, the medial epicondyles, and the lateral epicondyles. Ten to 12 thicknesses of splinting material should be wet with water, placed onto the posterior arm, and molded around the circumference. The arm should be held in the desired degree of flexion while the ace wrap is applied.

Sugar Tong Splint

The sugar tong splint covers the forearm from above the elbow to the metacarpal heads. It is used to temporarily immobilize wrist and forearm fractures. It prevents supinating and pronating of the forearm. This splint allows for post injury swelling. The patient's arm is measured from the volar metacarpal heads, around the elbow, to the dorsal metacarpal heads to determine the length of material needed. Eight to 10 layers of cast padding, and plaster, are laid out. The plaster is dipped, drained of excess water, and placed on top of the padding. The padding side is placed against the skin, and the splint wrapped around the arm. The volar and dorsal forearm is covered by the splint. The splint is wrapped with an ace wrap. The material surrounding the elbow must be folded smoothly, to ensure that pressure over the bony prominences is not increased.

Tennis Elbow Brace

Tennis elbow is the name commonly given to lateral epicondylitis. This condition involves inflammation of the tendons of the wrist extensors at the insertion point on the lateral elbow. Tennis elbow generally presents as pain at this site. An elbow brace can support the joint, and relieve pain in the area. This brace allows the wearer to remain active. It consists of a strap the goes around the proximal forearm. A pad is attached to the strap and this fits over the proximal muscle bellies of the wrist extensor muscles. This strap must be worn fairly tightly to support the tendons and provide pain relief. When the wrist extends, the area compressed by the pad serves as an anchor for muscle contraction. This relieves pressure where the tendon inserts on the elbow.

Bracing and Splinting for Carpal Tunnel Syndrome

Carpal tunnel syndrome is caused by the compression of the median nerve within the carpal tunnel of the wrist. The size of the tunnel decreases as the wrist is flexed, increasing compression. Efforts to treat the condition by bracing the wrist focus on preventing flexion. To this end, a cock-up, or carpal tunnel splint, is used. This type of splint holds the wrist in a neutral, or slightly extended, position which relieves pressure on the median nerve. As the brace is bulky and awkward, it is often worn only at night. This prevents the wearer from sleeping on the wrist while it is in a flexed position, and this prevents further irritation of the nerve. Bracing may not reduce symptoms significantly in severe cases of carpal tunnel syndrome, but in mild or moderate cases bracing may allow the avoidance of surgery.

Ulnar Gutter Splint

Ulnar gutter splints are often used to treat fractures of the metacarpals and phalanges of the ring and small fingers. The splint starts at the forearm and extends to the tip of the ring and small fingers. If the injury pattern warrants, the long finger is included in the splint. Fingers can be splinted using a traditional cast, or a pre-fabricated splint can be used. In either case, the casting material is wet down, placed onto the padding, and positioned on the ulnar side of the arm. It is then wrapped around the forearm, wrist, and hand. The fingers will be straight, or flexed to approximately 90 degrees at the metacarpal-phalangeal joints. A 2 inch ace wrap is used to fix the splint in place. The technologist holds the splint in position until it has dried and hardened.

Baseball, Airplane, Dynamic, and Co-Aptation Splints

A baseball splint is a prefabricated splint which is used to stabilize fractures of the distal phalanx. It is applied to the volar side of the hand and forearm. It is called a baseball splint as it positions the hand in such a way that it looks like a baseball is being held in the palm.

An airplane splint holds the arm in a position of abduction at shoulder level. The forearm is in flexion, and a strut is used for support.

A dynamic splint describes any kind of splint that uses springs, or elastic bands, to provide a constant force to control position and range of motion.

A co-aptation splint consists of 2 pads of plaster placed on either side of an extremity, and held in place by a dressing. Instead of 2 pads, 1 u-shaped pad may be used.

Sling and Swath for Proximal Humerus Fracture

Proximal humerus fractures often occur in the elderly as a result of a fall on an outstretched arm. A combined sling and swathe is often used to stabilize the injury, and ease pain. The first component of the brace is a standard sling. This is fitted to the patient and the strap crossing the neck is padded. The swathe component is added after the sling is fitted. A pre-fabricated swathe can be used, or a simple ace wrap. The swathe is wrapped around the patient's body and over the fractured humerus. The wrap must be tight, but not so tight to cause discomfort. Depending upon the severity of the fracture, the sling and swathe may be used without further treatment. If the fracture requires surgery, this splint can be used to make the patient more comfortable before surgery.

Finger Traps for Fracture Reductions

Simple displaced fractures of the wrist and hand can often be treated with reduction and casting. Finger traps may be used to make reduction easier. These devices involve metal or plastic sheaths that affix to the fingers of the affected hand. The patient lies face up on the examination table with the injured arm at the edge. The elbow is bent at a 90 degree angle while the hand and forearm hand are held vertically. The fingers traps are then placed on the fingers. A strap is positioned across the biceps of the injured arm to allow the addition of counterweight. This arrangement of traction/counter traction helps bring the bone fragments into proper alignment. The arm is kept in this position for several minutes to allow the muscles of the wrist to relax. Following reduction, a cast can be applied.

Velpeau Dressing/Sling

A Velpeau dressing, also called a Velpeau sling, is designed to treat injuries to the shoulder and humerus. It can be used to treat fractures, or dislocations in these areas. This device is used when the fracture is minimally displaced, or nondisplaced. It is similar to a sling and swathe dressing, but it more restrictive. The elbow is held at the side in a flexed position, and the hand is affixed to the upper chest. It is generally used to treat injuries in individuals who would not be able to tolerate other kinds of treatment. It is therefore often used to treat young children, or the elderly. The angulation of the fracture can be controlled by pads placed in the axilla.

Hinged Brace Treatment for Isolated Medial Collateral Ligament Injuries

The medial collateral ligament (MCL) is located on the medial side of the knee joint and extends from the femur to the tibia. This ligament stops the knee from moving away from the midline of the body. A torn MCL results in an unstable knee joint. Patients with MCL tears should be checked for meniscal tears; they are often associated. Conservative treatment is directed at increasing knee stability. Most isolated MCL tears can be treated without surgery as the ligament will form scar tissue and heal, restoring stability to the joint. The use of a hinged knee brace is usually advised to promote the healing process. The brace is fitted to the knee and features rigid fixation along the lateral and medial sides. The brace has hinges built into both sides to permit the knee joint to flex and extend while preventing movement inward, or outward. Frequent adjustments may be required initially to ensure adequate stability.

Knee Unloader Braces for Degenerative Conditions

The incidence of degenerative arthritis of the knee is increasing with the increase in activity level in society. When the cartilage in the knee degenerates, the underlying bone loses its cushion, and the ensuing friction leads to pain. Most approaches to addressing this pain are invasive (injections and surgery), or require the continuing use of medication. The unloader brace is a non-invasive therapy. It is often the case that one side of the knee is degenerative (usually the medial), and one side is healthy. To balance this, the unloader brace puts pressure on the healthy side of the knee with counter pressure above and below the damaged side. This creates a triangle of support with the base of the triangle on the affected side. This serves to correct the misalignment of the knee, restore function, and decrease pain. Multiple fittings of the brace may be required.

Patellar Brace for PFC

In patellar femoral chondromalacia (PFC) the cartilage under the patella becomes damaged. Extension and flexion of the knee causes pain as the patella rubs against the femur. This condition may result from a muscle imbalance in the quadriceps that causes the patella to be pulled laterally preventing it from sliding smoothly in the groove of the femur. Exercises to strengthen the medial side of the quadriceps may aid in pulling the patella over. The use of a patellar brace will often be advised until the muscular imbalance is resolved. This brace is fitted over the knee and has a large pad on the lateral side that pushes the patella toward the midline into proper alignment. The correct fitting and sizing of these braces is imperative because the pad must fit precisely along the lateral patella.

Patellar Tendonitis

The patella tendon extends from the inferior border of the patella to the tibial tubercle. This tendon is involved in knee extension. Inflammation of this tendon can occur as a result of repetitive activities, or strain. Patellar tendonitis, also called jumper's knee, is a painful condition. Rest, ice, and anti-inflammatory drugs are the usual treatment for patellar tendonitis, but if complete rest until the problem has resolved is not possible, bracing may be beneficial. A brace for this condition is composed of an elastic knee sleeve with an open area at the patella. Another support device is a patellar strap which is worn across the body of the tendon. This strap is reasonably comfortable, and will allow resumption of activities.

Extension Bracing for Spinal Compression Fractures

Spinal compression fractures, also called vertebral compression fractures, can occur as a result of trauma, osteoporosis, infection, or cancer. In a compression fracture, the vertebra collapses and takes up a smaller space in the vertebral column. This compression shows up as a loss of vertebral height on x-rays. Treatment may involve surgery, or extension bracing. Spinal compression causes the forward flexion of the body at the site of the fracture. Extension bracing helps to prevent this. An extension brace consists of a rigid brace worn below the level of the fracture, and a rigid pad which applies pressure across the patient's chest. This device helps keep the body in an appropriate position to allow healing. In some cases, surgery is indicated.

Lace Up Ankle Braces

The taping of ankles to treat and prevent injuries is a common practice among athletes during sports activities. Studies have shown, however, tape quickly stretches and loosens decreasing its supportive properties and benefits. A lace up ankle brace made from nylon webbing is a useful alternative to taping the ankle. The tightness of the brace can be controlled. The brace can be laced to provide the desired level of support. This is superior to taping as a brace can be tightened, or loosened, as required while tape must be removed in order to adjust its support level. Bracing is a less expensive alternative in the long run as new supplies do not need to be bought on a continuing basis. A brace can be cleaned and reused unlike tape.

AFO

An Ankle Foot Orthosis (AFO) is a brace that holds the foot in a neutral position. It accomplishes this by preventing plantar flexion. The AFO starts at the proximal calf and continues along the planter surface of the foot. This device is very useful in the treatment of a drop foot injury in which the nerves to the foot's dorsiflexor muscles are damaged. The dorsiflexor muscles are used in normal walking to lift the foot, and ensure that the heel strikes the ground before the toes. Individuals with a case of drop foot that goes untreated often stub their toes which may cause falls. AFOs can be purchased off the shelf, but a custom made brace is more efficient, and therefore preferable. A technologist may be involved in the fitting of the AFO brace.

Compression Devices

The hands, fingers, and thumb are susceptible to injury involving swelling and impaired functioning. Treatment for fractures and soft tissue injuries in these areas should be followed up by measures to decrease swelling. Initially, efforts are made to improve range of motion in the hand and digits with physical therapy. The technologist should assist the patient in the use of compression devices to work in conjunction with this therapy. Compression devices include ace wraps, or tubular stockings, which are designed to completely enclose the damaged area. Compression helps push the excess fluid out of the limb, and back into systemic circulation. Compression devices should be snug, but not so snug as to impair of the neurovascular functioning.

Crutches

Crutches are used to take the weight off of an injured lower extremity. The use of crutches requires walking with short even strides. The crutches are help near the body, and the weight is borne by the hands and arms. A distance of 3 fingers should be kept between the armpit, and the top of the crutch. There are 4 types of gaits possible when using crutches. In the step-through gait, the injured leg is moved forward followed by the uninjured leg. In the two- point gait, the injured leg, and the crutches move together, and the uninjured leg follows. In the three-point gait, each crutch, and the uninjured leg move separately. The four-point gait involves each crutch and each leg moving separately.

Traction

TRACTION

Traction is the application of a pulling force in the treatment of skeletal and muscular disorders, or abnormalities. It is generally used for disorders of the extremities, vertebral column, or pelvis. Traction is used in the treatment of many types of disorders, including dislocations, fractures, and muscle spasms. It may be used short-term, or for longer periods of time. Traction is used to bring the fragments of a fracture into alignment, to ease pain, and to ease muscle spasms. Although there are 2 main types of traction (skeletal, and skin), there are many forms of these traction types designed to treat particular injuries, and disorders. The type of traction used depends upon the injury, and the age and health of the patient. Certain medical conditions rule out the use of certain methods of traction.

SKIN TRACTION

Skin traction involves the use of weights attached to the skin by various devices. The weights involved range from 5 – 7 pounds. Skin traction is preferred in cases where only light weights are required as it is noninvasive. The weights are attached to the skin by means of tape, straps, boots, or cuffs. The skin attachment devices must be loose enough to allow proper circulation. Injuries requiring the use of heavy weights cannot be treated with skin traction, as the skin will not hold up, and will slough off. Skin traction is usually applied while the patient is in a hospital bed. There are numerous types of skin traction designed to treat particular injuries, or disorders.

BUCK'S TRACTION

Buck's traction is a type of skin traction. It provides longitudinal traction on an extremity by means of an apparatus involving adhesive tape attached to the skin. A cord attached to the adhesive tape is fed through a pulley. A weight is attached the other end of the cord to provide necessary tension. Today, a special splint is often used in place of adhesive tape. This splint has external Velcro straps which allow it to be tightened as necessary. The use of a splint is easier on the patient's skin than the traditional method using adhesive tape. Buck's traction is commonly used to treat patients with fractures who are waiting to undergo a surgical procedure.

DISADVANTAGES

Buck's traction would be an inappropriate form of treatment in a number of cases. Extensive soft tissue injury would rule out this form of traction as it would be painful and could exacerbate the damage to the tissue. The pressure exerted in this form of traction could cause ischemic changes in patients with poor peripheral circulation. Long term use of this technique could lead to skin shearing and the development of pressure sores. The technique itself limits the amount of weight that can be used for traction; some injuries require more weight than can be supported using Buck's traction. For example, fractures of the acetabulum frequently require traction of the lower leg to reduce the force of the femoral head on the fracture site. This requires more weight than can be used with Buck's traction. For these fractures traction is usually supplied by internal fixation.

RUSSELL'S TRACTION AND HARE TRACTION

Russell's traction is a type of skin traction. It uses skin traction on the lower leg to suspend the distal thigh by means of a sling. It is considered an improvement on Buck's traction. Split Russell's traction is often used to treat fractured hips in the elderly.

Hare traction is a form of temporary traction used while transporting acute injury cases. It is used in the field to treat fractured femurs. It realigns the ends of the fracture reducing pain, and restoring blood circulation. This treatment decreases the risk of further damage to nerves and tissues in the area. The splint consists of a long leg splint, a ratchet device to allow adjustment, and straps to help immobilize the leg.

Skeletal Traction

Skeletal traction is an invasive procedure that uses hardware placed in the bones. These pins, or screws, are applied during a surgical procedure under anesthetic. Skeletal is used when larger amounts of weight are required than can be used with skin traction. Larger weights mean more pulling force. This type of traction allows the use of 25 – 40 pound weights. The placement of the pins, or screws, must be accurate. This hardware can be left in the bones for a number of months. To prevent infection, the hardware and the area surrounding it must be kept clean. Although minor infections can be treated with antibiotics, more serious infections will require removal of the pins. The hardware may cause inflammation of the bone. Different types of skeletal traction have been developed to treat different injuries, and disorders. Patients requiring skeletal traction are generally immobilized for an extended length of time.

Bryant's Traction

Bryant's traction is used to maintain alignment of femoral fractures in children up to 2 years of age, or those weighing less than 30 lbs. Bryant's traction involves the use of compressive wraps wound around the leg. A rope extends from the wrap to the traction weight. Longitudinal traction is then applied and pulls the femoral head distally. Modified Bryant's traction is used in the reduction of congenital hip dislocations in young children. Congenital hip dislocations are often associated with tightness of the soft tissues surrounding the hip joint. This tightness makes reduction of the hip joint more difficult. The tightness of the surrounding tissue must be addressed. This traction is maintained for a period of time to gently stretch the soft tissues around the hip. Reduction is attempted once the hip joint is considered mobile enough.

Traction in Fracture Care

The muscles surrounding a fracture of a long bone may contract, and displace the major fragments. This causes malalignment of the joint, swelling, and increased pain. This displacement can also cause increased pressure on nerves, or blood vessels, which can lead to irreversible damage to soft tissues distal to the fracture. Traction is used as a temporizing measure to correct the alignment of the fractured bone fragments, and take pressure off of the soft tissues surrounding the fracture. Traction exerts a force along the long axis of the bone by means of external fixation (splints, or adhesives), or internal fixation (pins). Traction often dramatically reduces the pain caused by the injury. The patient can be kept in traction until surgical fixation can be performed. In rare cases where the patient is unable to tolerate surgery, traction may be used on its own to allow healing.

Dunlop's Traction

Dunlop's traction is most frequently used to treat supracondylar elbow fractures in children. This method helps maintain the reduction, and helps prevent neurovascular compromise. Dunlop's traction most often involves skin traction, but it is can also involve a combination of skin and skeletal traction. The patient is positioned face up in the hospital bed with the affected extremity positioned at the edge of the bed. This form of traction works by applying weight traction at the distal end of the humerus, and counteracting this with longitudinal traction of the forearm. The forearm traction must hold the elbow at a 90 degree angle. Continuing neurovascular examinations should be conducted during traction.

Surgery

General Information to Report to the Surgeon Regarding a Fracture

The surgeon needs to know the location of the fracture. This covers what bone is broken and where on the bone the fracture is located. The surgeon might be told, for example, that the patient has a right femur, mid-shaft fracture. The next point to consider is whether the fracture is open or closed. An open fracture is one in which the broken bone has pierced the skin. This is a serious condition as it could lead to a significant infectious process. Any fracture involving a skin injury should be treated as open until proven otherwise. The third piece of information needed by the surgeon is the type of fracture present.

After describing the location and severity of the fracture, its anatomical alignment should be described. The surgeon should be told whether the broken bone is still in its normal position, or if it is displaced. The distal fragment of a fractured bone can also be at an angle to the proximal fragment. This is called the angulation of the fracture. The degree angulation will be of particular concern to the surgeon. The final step in describing a fracture involves the neurovascular status of the limb. The lack of a pulse, or disruption in the nerve function distal to the fracture is a medical emergency, and the orthopedic surgeon must be alerted to these situations immediately.

Surgical Hand Washing Procedure

Remove all jewelry, and examine fingers, hands, and forearms for sites of skin damage, and soiling. Use a nail pick to clean under each fingernail. After obtaining a sterile scrub brush, start the water and wet the arms to a site 2 inches above the elbow. Clean 1 arm at a time with 30 passes in each area. Scrub under the nails using the rough side of the scrub brush. Clean the dorsal, radial, ulnar, and volar sides of the finger. Scrub the palm and dorsal hand surfaces. Scrub the 4 sides of the forearm. Extend the scrub to 2 inches above the elbow. Repeat the process for the opposite arm. Holding the hands higher than the elbows, rinse each arm from the fingertips back toward the elbow. Excess water should be allowed to drip into the sink.

Attire

The operating room contains a semirestricted and restricted area. Different attire is required depending upon the function of the wearer. These types of attire are as follows: OR attire, protective attire, and scrub (sterile) attire. Certain types of attire are worn by all personnel entering the operating room, and some types are worn only by individuals performing specific jobs. Hair covering, for example is a part of OP attire, but is also considered as protective attire. Each health care facility has a written policy outlining the type of attire to be worn for each job. All individuals involved in the surgical procedure go through the nonrestricted area to the locker room to change into attire acceptable for their position in the operating room.

Protective Attire

Protective attire is worn to protect the staff member and patient from microbes, and environmental hazards such as radiation and lasers. Protective attire includes the scrub suit, mask, hair cover, shoe covers, nonsterile gloves, protective eyewear, and radiation protection. Nonsterile gloves are required any time contact with bodily fluids, may occur. Nonsterile gloves come in latex and vinyl. If the patient, or staff member, is allergic to latex, nylons gloves must be worn. Clean objects should not be touched with soiled gloves, and gloves should be discarded after use. Protective eyewear must be worn whenever exposure to body fluids is likely. The eye is a primary site for exposure to blood borne disease. Eyewear, or shields, should cover the eyes from all sides. Radiation protection methods include portable lead screens, lead aprons, lead sternal/thyroid shields, leaded glasses, and lead-impregnated gloves.

Attire Worn in the OR

Special attire is worn in these areas of the OR to limit microbial spread. Attire always worn in the operating room includes the scrub suit, and hair cover. Mask, and shoe covers may be required. After each use, the scrubs are laundered. Although scrubs are often worn by personnel after leaving the surgical services area, scrubs soiled by blood, and body fluids should be changed right away, to prevent cross contamination. In some facilities scrubs must be changed upon leaving the surgical services area. A cap, or hood, is worn to cover hair on the head, and sides of the face. Head covers come in disposable and non-disposable types. Masks are used to protect sterile supplies from contamination by the staff, and to protect the staff from inhaled contaminants. Shoe covers are worn primarily to protect personnel against contamination by bodily fluids during surgery.

Scrub (Sterile) Attire

Scrub attire is worn by the surgical team. This attire is put on after the surgical scrub. It consists of the sterile gown, and sterile gloves. This attire is sterile, and is required for entry into the sterile field of surgery. The surgical gown is made of woven, or nonwoven, fabric that is lint-free. Only part of the gown is considered sterile. The sterile part of the gown includes the front section from mid-chest to waist, and the front part of the sleeves. The cuffs of the gown are not considered sterile, and must be covered by the gloves. Sterile gloves are put on after the gown. There are a number of types of gloves which have been developed for the different surgical specialties. Double-gloving, wearing 2 sets of gloves is recommended.

Double-Gloving

Double-gloving provides extra protection from injury and disease. Diseases are less likely to be transmitted through a puncture wound to the hand if the hand has been double-gloved. This is because as the sharp object passes through the glove material, biological material (bioburden) is removed. This leaves less biological material to enter the wound. There are several other reasons for double-gloving. Fat breaks down latex, allowing passage of contaminants. The ability of latex to act as a barrier decreases over time. As latex gloves contain spaces, they may become saturated with blood and other bodily fluids. This can create passageways through the gloves which allow the fluids to reach the skin of the wearer. When wearing 2 gloves, a glove of a larger size than is normally worn is worn next to the skin, and a glove of normal size is worn on top.

Body Exhaust Suits During Total Joint Replacements

Total joint replacement surgery involves the resurfacing, or reconstructing, of a degenerative joint using a metallic implant. An implant is a potential location of infection. Infection of a total joint prosthesis may have adverse consequences in terms of function, mobility and patient mortality. The body exhaust suit, worn by members of the surgical team, was developed to prevent infection. The helmet of this suit has a closed shield which fits over the head. This suit prevents the team member from exhaling potentially contagious particles into the surgical field. A battery powered fan in the helmet circulates air within the helmet to prevent overheating. The suit also protects the wearer from the patient's bodily fluids. Joint replacement surgery involves techniques which could cause blood and tissue to become airborne. The full face shield prevents this tissue from contacting the skin and eyes of the surgical team members.

Supine Position

In the supine position, the patient is positioned flat on the back, with the arms secured at the sides of the body, palms facing inward. The legs are positioned straight out, so that the vertebrae are in a straight line with the hips. A safety belt is positioned across the thighs approximately 2 inches above the knees. If arm boards are used, these are positioned so that the arm is at no more than a 90 degree angle to the table. This is to ensure that the shoulder is not hyperextended. The elbows may be padded. Pillows may be placed under the head, and the curve of the lumbar spine. Bony sites of the body in contact with the table should be padded. A pillow, or padded footboard, may be used to support the feet so that they are not in plantar flexion for a prolonged period of time.

Fowler's Position

Fowler's position is a modified supine position. It provides better access to certain surgical sites than the supine position. This position decreases blood circulation to the upper body, and encourages venous drainage. An air embolism is a potential hazard of the position. Fowler's position allows easy access to the breast, head and neck, and shoulder. Before being placed in Fowler's position, the patient is placed in the supine position. A padded foot rest is attached to the operating table. The arms are secured across the stomach on a pillow, or on armboards. The hips are placed at the bend of the table. The lower section of the table is lowered. The upper section of the table is raised so that it is at a 45 degree angle. The whole table is then tilted downward to the desired level. Pressure points should be protected with padding.

Prone Position

The patient is anesthetized before being placed on the operating table in the prone position. The body regions which can be reached with the patient in this position include the posterior lower limb, the dorsal surface of the body, the spine, and the posterior cranium. Pads are applied as needed to the bony prominences of the knees ankles, and elbows. Chest rolls are positioned. The head is either turned to the side to rest on a pillow, or positioned face down to rest on a special head rest. The arms are secured along the length of the body with the palms facing upward, or toward the body. Alternatively, the arms may be positioned on armboards so that the palms face downward. A pillow is positioned under the patient's ankles. The safety strap is applied on the thighs, above the knees.

Beach Chair Positioning for Shoulder Surgery

The patient is placed on the table, and after induction of anesthesia the back of the chair is raised to a slightly reclined sitting position. The patient's lower back must be positioned against the chair to avoid damage. The neck and head should be put in a neutral position, and a towel placed across the forehead. The head should then be fixed to the head rest of the table by taping across the towel. This will prevent damage to the skin and eyebrows. The non-operative arm should be positioned on a padded arm board so that the bony prominences are protected. The medial epicondylar region is of particular concern due to possible injury to the ulnar nerve. Posteriorly, the draping should hug the medial border of the scapula. Anteriorly, draping must be medial to the coracoid process. The top drape should hug the mid clavicle.

Lateral Position

The lateral position is also called the lateral recumbent position, and the lateral decubitus position. The patient is positioned on one side, with the opposite side of the body facing upward. The areas of the body that can be accessed include the retroperitoneal space, the hip, and the hemithorax. Before being placed in the lateral position, the patient is placed in the supine position. Padding is used on the ankles, knees, and elbows. The patient is then rolled onto the side in question. The head is stabilized with a pillow. The lower leg is flexed, and two pillows are positioned between the legs. The upper leg is left straight. A safety strap is positioned over the hip. The shoulders and spine are put into alignment. The arms are placed on double armboards with the palm of the lower arm facing upward, and the palm of the upper arm facing downward.

Anterior Cruciate Ligament Reconstruction Positioning

Proper positioning is extremely important for achieving a successful outcome in ACL reconstruction surgery. The tourniquet must be placed as proximally as possible on the thigh of the affected leg. A leg holder, or lateral post, attached to the bed by brackets on the side rails is used to hold the leg in position for surgery. Proper positioning places the patient's knee at the break in the table. This permits the extremity in question to be flexed to at least 90 degrees for surgery. The other leg should be well padded to protect it from injury. The leg is draped after prepping. The thigh proximal to the knee must be exposed to allow for bone tunnel and graft placement. Improper draping and positioning may lead to a lack of sufficient room for these. This may result in the guide pin exiting the thigh and entering a non-sterile area contaminating the field.

Fracture Table for Positioning to Repair Hip and Femur Fractures

Fractures of the hip and femur often displace as a result of tension from the thigh and groin muscles attached to the bone. Without direct muscular opposition, the bone fragments get pulled in opposite directions. Fractures of the hip and thigh require surgical treatment using open reduction internal fixation, or intra-medullary rodding. A standard operating table is not appropriate for these procedures because these techniques require maintained traction. The fracture table allows the necessary traction to be maintained. The fracture table includes a boot which is fixed to a mobile post by a bracket. The foot on the affected leg is placed in this boot. The bracket has a winch that ensures the desired tension is maintained on the muscles. The non-operative leg is placed in a leg holder to keep the hip flexed, and away from the patient's midline to allow imaging studies of the injured leg.

Lateral Positioner for Hip Replacement/Hemi-Arthroplasty Surgery

The lateral hip positioner, used in hip replacement surgery and bipolar hemi-arthroplasty, allows the patient to be firmly secured during the procedure, and provides a stable platform on which to operate. The patient is turned so that he/she is lying on the non-operative side. The posterior positioner is then put into use. This apparatus consists of a pad that locks into place with a bracket that attaches to the table. The pad should be positioned so that it lies in the center of the patient's lumbar spine at the L4-L5 level. The anterior pad, also affixed to the table via brackets, is then pressed closely to the anterior superior iliac spine. The positioning must allow the operative leg to be flexed to 90 degrees for the femoral stem placement. All bony prominences should be well padded to avoid nerve injuries.

Surgical Drapes

Surgical drapes are used to protect the surgical site from contamination that could cause an infection. The drapes used in surgery act as a physical barrier that prevents microorganisms from moving to the sterile environment. Drape material should not contain lint, as this can provide airborne particles with a way into the wound. Drapes should be fluid resistant to stop strike-through contamination of the surgical wound. Drapes must be antistatic to ensure sparking does not occur. Drapes should be strong, and not easily torn. Surgical drapes must be porous so that the patient does not suffer hyperthermia from retained body heat. The color of drapes must not reflect the operating lights, as this could interfere with vision. Drapes must be flame retardant. Finally, drapes must be free of any toxins. Drapes may be made from woven textile fabric, nonwoven textile fabric, and plastic. Different materials have different advantages and disadvantages.

Plastic Drapes

There are 2 types of plastic adhesive drapes. These are incise drapes, and aperture drapes. Incise drapes are made of thin see-through plastic. They have an adhesive back. These drapes are applied on top of folded towels. The surgical incision is made through the drape while it is on the patient. Aperture drapes are made of clear plastic. The fenestrations of these drapes are surrounded by adhesive backing. The clear plastic allows the surgeon to see landmarks that would be covered by other drapes. Small aperture drapes are often used to drape the eyes. Isolation aperture drapes are large, and are often used for surgery requiring pinning of the hip.

Woven Textile Fabric and Nonwoven Textile Fabric Drapes

Nonwoven textile fabrics are disposable, light, and strong. They are made from synthetic materials. They do not need to be washed and sterilized and folded, so there is little chance of contamination. Reinforced layers of material surround the fenestration (opening). Woven textile fabrics are reusable. They are becoming popular because it is cheaper to launder them than to replace disposable drapes. The material swells when wet, and becomes impermeable. Woven textile fabric drapes are treated with a fluorochemical to increase their fluid repellant nature. The disadvantages of these drapes are that they must be washed, sterilized, inspected for damage, and repaired. Small holes can be missed. Holes compromise the drape's function as a barrier.

Fenestrated Drapes

Fenestrated drapes have openings to expose the site of the surgical incision. Each type of drape is suited for a type of surgery. Drape types have a fenestration of a particular shape, in a particular place, depending upon their intended use. A laparotomy drape has a large, long fenestration in the middle to allow exposure for an incision on the abdomen. The remainder of the drape should be large enough to provide cover for the feet, and anesthesia screen. If the fenestrated drape is not long enough, a nonfenestrated drape may be added. Fenestrated sheets are used for procedures on the following sections of anatomy: abdomen, thorax and kidney, neck, arms and legs, hips, perineum, and cranium.

Nonfenestrated Drapes

Nonfenestrated sheets are used to cover sections not covered by the fenestrated sheet, or for custom draping. Flat sheets are a type of nonfenestrated drape. They are square, or rectangular, sheets. They may be used under an arm, or leg. Flat drapes may also be used to cover arms on an armboard. Nonfenestrated drapes are also custom made for surgeries on specific areas of the body. One end of a nonfenestrated split sheet is open down the middle. These sheets are used to drape extremities, or to create an opening at a surgical incision site. The nonfenestrated split sheet has a U shape, and the free ends of the sheet are called the tails.

Sterile Packs

Sterile packs are designed for medical specialties, and for specific procedures. For example, there are specific packs for orthopedic surgeries, and there are specific packs for arthroscopic procedures. The packs contain the required supplies for the particular specialty, or procedure. Basic packs generally contain a Mayo stand cover, 2 surgical gowns, a suture bag, 4 sticky paper drapes, and 2 paper towels. The required type of drapes and specialty supplies are added to the packs to customize them. A customized pack may be requested by an institution, and prepared by a manufacturer. Some sterile packs are prepared by the institution using reusable supplies. The sterile packs are opened and used as the initial sterile field.

Stockinette Drapes

Stockinette drapes are stretchy tubes designed to cover the arms and legs. One end of the tube is open, and the other is closed. The closed end of the tube covers the distal part of the extremity, and the open end of the tube covers the proximal part of the extremity. The stockinette drape is contained in a pre-packaged roll, and is unrolled over the extremity. The arm, or leg, is held up to allow the stockinette to be positioned correctly. The stockinette may be covered with plastic to make it impermeable to fluids. Stockinettes are often used to cover the arms and legs in coronary bypass surgeries, or hip replacement surgeries.

General Anesthesia

General anesthesia produces a change in level of consciousness, and level of perception. It is used for extensive procedures, or for procedures that need a higher level of anesthesia than regional anesthesia can provide. The agents used to produce general anesthesia are administered by injection, instillation, or inhalation. Agent injection generally involves the introduction of medications directly into the blood stream, but some medications may be injected intramuscularly. Agent instillation involves the introduction of a medication into an area where it can be absorbed through the mucous membranes. Agent inhalation involves the introduction of gases to the alveolar membrane where they are absorbed into the vascular system. The agents circulate through the body. General anesthesia suppresses coughing, gagging, breathing, and other protective reflexes. Because of this, the use of general anesthesia also requires the use of breathing aids such as a tube.

Local Anesthesia

Local anesthesia is produced by the injection of an agent that blocks nerve conduction into the tissues around a peripheral nerve. This type of anesthesia blocks pain in a specific area of the body. It does not affect alertness. The anesthetic agent can produce anesthesia within 5-15 minutes. The duration of the anesthesia produced depends upon the anesthetic agent used. The effectiveness of the agent may be prolonged by the addition of epinephrine, or hyaluronidase. The administration of more anesthetic may be necessary after the initial dose if the site of surgery is enlarged, or if additional layers of tissue become involved. This type of anesthesia is used for such things as skin biopsies, or stitches in the skin. Some types of frequently used injectable local anesthetics include procaine, lidocaine, and tetracaine.

Topical Anesthesia

Anesthesia involves the use an agent that blocks nerve conduction. A topical anesthesia is one that blocks nerve conduction after being placed directly on a tissue layer, such as the skin, or mucous membrane. The only area anesthetized is the area in direct contact with the anesthetic agent. The onset of the anesthetic effect is rapid. The duration of the effect depends upon the particular agent, and the dose administered. Topical anesthesia is used to anesthetize the mucous membranes of the upper aerodigestive tract, the urethra, the vagina, the rectum, and the skin. Topical anesthesia is achieved by means of cryoanesthesia, or a pharmaceutical agent. Cryoanesthesia uses localized cooling to reduce nerve conduction. This cooling may be produced by ice, a cryoanesthesia machine, or a localized freeze spray. Pharmaceutical agents used to produce topical anesthesia are absorbed through the skin, and come into contact with peripheral nerve endings.

Conscious Sedation

Conscious sedation is also called intravenous sedation. It is used to induce relaxation, and sleepiness. It involves the administration of pain medication, and a mild sedative intravenously. As a side effect, this type of sedation causes temporary forgetfulness, and the patient may not recall events that occurred during the surgical procedure. Although conscious sedation may cause forgetfulness, the patient is awake enough to respond to questions posed during the procedure. Protective reflexes, such as swallowing, or coughing are unaffected. If secretions accumulate, the patient can cough, or swallow to clear them. Conscious sedation is often used for such procedures as colonoscopies. Conscious sedation may be used in combination with regional anesthesia.

Regional Anesthesia

Regional anesthesia is produced by the administration of an anesthetic along a major nerve tract. It is used to block the sensation of pain in a region of the body. Regional anesthesia blocks nerve conduction from all tissues distal to the site of injection. Regional anesthesia does not cause loss of consciousness, or loss of alertness. This type of anesthesia has a slower onset of action than local anesthesia. The duration of action is agent dependent. There are different types of regional anesthesia, including spinal block, and epidural block. Regional anesthesia is very effective in producing anesthesia in selected areas, while leaving other areas unaffected. This type of anesthesia can also decrease postoperative pain.

Nerve Plexus Block

A nerve plexus block involves the injection of an anesthetic agent into the site of a major plexus. Examples of nerve plexus blocks are injections into the brachial plexus, or the cervical plexus. The tissue affected by the anesthetic agent includes all the tissue innervated by the plexus. A nerve plexus block is often used in conjunction with intravenous sedation. A nerve plexus block has less impact on the system than general anesthesia, but still allows the anesthetic to have an effect during the immediate postoperative and recovery phase. This type of nerve block has surgical, diagnostic, and therapeutic uses. It can also be used to determine the prognosis of a permanent intervention.

Spinal Block

A spinal block is also called an intrathecal block. It involves an injection of an anesthetic agent into the cerebral spinal fluid surrounding the spinal cord. The anesthetic is injected in a single dose. A spinal block causes loss of sensation to the body below the diaphragm, and a loss of muscle control. The onset of the effect of a spinal block is quick, occurring in 3-10 minutes. The duration of this form of anesthesia depends upon the anesthetic used but is generally 1-1 ½ hours. The duration of the anesthetic may be prolonged by use of an additive to the anesthetic. As patient cooperation is essential to this procedure, a sedative is usually given first.

Epidural Block

An epidural block involves the injection of an anesthetic agent into the epidural space between the vertebrae. This is inside the spinal canal, but outside the dura. Although epidurals may be administered in any spinal region, spinal blocks are generally administered in the neck, or lower back. Epidurals are rarely used in the thoracic spine. The epidural space contains spinal cord, and spinal nerves. The anesthetic is injected in such a manner as to spread out and cover all the nerve roots in the area of injection. In the administration of an epidural, a local anesthetic is given via a small needle to numb the site, and then the epidural needle is inserted.

Bier Block

A Bier block is method of administering a regional anesthetic to an extremity. It delivers the anesthetic intravenously. This technique involves the use of a double tourniquet. The blood is squeezed out of the limb, and prevented from returning to the limb. The anesthetic is then injected directly into the vein. The tourniquet prevents the anesthetic from leaving the extremity, and prevents blood from entering the extremity. It also gives the surgeon a surgical field clear of blood. This method of anesthesia is easy, and provides the surgeon with a clear operating field. There is a time limit to its use however, due to the restriction of blood flow to the area. Surgery must be completed in 1 -2 hours. Te tourniquet must not be removed before sufficient anesthetic has been metabolized, or toxic amounts may be released into the bloodstream.

Axillary Block

The axillary block is a regional anesthetic. It involves the injection of an anesthetic agent into the nerves surrounding the axillary artery. It is useful surgeries involving the hand and forearm. To administer this block in the adult, the patient is positioned so that the arm is abducted, and is flexed at the elbow to form a 90 degree angle. The axillary artery is palpated as high up in the axilla as possible. The needle is then inserted to the side of the artery. The effects of the anesthetic will last 4 - 18 hours depending upon the medication, and amount of medication, used. This method of anesthesia may produce a painful bruise.

Interscalene Block

An interscalene block is a regional anesthetic. It involves the injection of anesthetic between the scalene muscles of the neck. It is used to provide anesthesia during medical procedures on the arm, and shoulder. It is a very useful form of anesthetic for the upper part of the extremity, but is less efficient in blocking nerves in the hand and wrist. It can be used to block cervical nerves, and nerves in the brachial plexus. The brachial plexus innervates the shoulder. The block can last from 4 - 18 hours depending upon the amount of anesthetic administered. A nerve stimulator is often used to help guide the needle into the proper site. The nerve stimulator will cause twitches in the muscles it is being used to stimulate. This will be used to ascertain if the needle is in the right spot before the anesthetic is administered.

Elbow Blocks, Wrist Blocks, Digital Blocks, and Transthecal Blocks

Elbow blocks, wrist blocks, digital blocks, and transthecal blocks are all methods of regional anesthesia, and all involve the injection of anesthetic agents. An elbow block is a rarely used method of anesthesia for procedures on the upper limbs. They are sometimes used in conjunction with axillary blocks. A wrist block is a common form of anesthesia for procedures on the hand. Wrist blocks without another type of anesthesia are used for procedures that last less than 30 minutes. A digital block is the most common method of anesthesia used for procedures on the hand. The nerves of the digits can be blocked on the dorsal side, and/or volar side of the hand. A transthecal block is used to anesthetize the digits. The anesthetic is injected into the flexor sheath.

Monitored Anesthesia Care

Monitored anesthesia care is also known as MAC. It involves the use of local, or topical, nerve conduction blocks, combined with the use of analgesics, sedatives, or amnesiacs. The analgesics, sedatives, and amnesiacs are generally administered as inhalants, or by injection. The dosages of the analgesics, sedatives, or amnesiacs are low enough that patient ventilation is not required during surgery. Although sedated and in a light sleep, the patient is able to respond if requested to do so. By the end of the procedure, the patient is awake. Although this type of care is often used for individuals with complex medical problems, MAC is also used as a supplement to local and regional anesthesia. The patient may request this type of care. MAC requires the participation of an anesthesiologist as well as a surgeon.

Surgical Sponges

There are many different kinds of surgical sponge. These include laparotomy sponges, Raytech sponges, neurosurgical sponges, tonsil sponges, Kitner dissecting sponges, and peanut sponges. Surgical sponges have many uses in surgical procedures. They are used to absorb bodily fluids, such as blood. They can be used in the blunt dissection of tissue. Surgical sponges are also used as barriers to keep structures from being damaged during the surgical procedure. Surgical sponges are soft, and free of lint. They have a radiopaque strip so that they can be located by radiograph should they become lost in the body. Surgical sponges are usually counted, to ensure that they are not left behind after surgery.

Laparotomy Sponges, Raytec Sponges, and Neurosurgical Sponges

Laparotomy sponges are the largest of the surgical sponges, and are the most absorbent. They are commonly called laps, tapes, or packs. They come in a number of sizes. They are used in procedures that involve large incisions. They are generally moistened with saline, and placed in such a way to protect the viscera. Raytec sponges are also called radiopaque four-by-fours. Raytec sponges are smaller than laparotomy sponges, and less absorbent. They are used for procedures requiring smaller incisions. Raytec sponges may be folded and attached to ring clamps to make sponge sticks for sponging and retracting within the incision. Raytec sponges are easily lost, and precautions must be taken to ensure that Raytec sponges are not left within the wound.

Neurological Sponges, Tonsil Sponges, Kitner Dissection Sponges, and Peanut Sponges

Neurosurgical sponges are also called patties, and cottonoids. They are used during neurological procedures to protect neural tissue, and to control bleeding. Neurosurgical sponges are used moistened with saline. Tonsil sponges are used in tonsillectomies. They are made of cotton filled gauze, and have a string attached. Tonsil sponges are used to pack the site after the removal of the tonsils. Kitner dissecting sponges are used in the blunt dissection of tissues. These sponges consist of small rolls of cotton tape. These sponges are always used attached to a clamp. Peanut sponges are small and made of gauze. They are used to blunt dissect tissue, or to absorb fluids. Peanut sponges are used with a clamp.

External Fixation vs. Open Reduction/Internal Fixation

External fixation and open reduction/internal fixation both have their uses. An external fixator is a frame that is used outside the body. It is attached to the bone by pins which pass through the skin via small incisions. These pins are placed in positions proximal and distal to the fracture site. External fixation permits the repair of the fracture without the disruption of the soft tissue overlying the fracture site. This can be beneficial to the healing process. External fixation can be particularly useful in cases involving open fractures, or those involving injuries with a great deal of damage to the soft tissue. An external fixation is generally a shorter procedure than an open reduction/internal fixation. An external fixator may be used to temporarily immobilize the fracture to allow time to develop a surgical plan, or to allow the patient to stabilize before surgery.

Limitations of External Fixators

The fixation supplied by external fixators is not as rigid as that supplied by internal hardware. This could result in the displacement of the reduction. Also, it is difficult to combine casting, or splinting, with the use of external fixators. Of great concern is the possibility of infection at the pin sites. The external fixator attaches to the bone by means of pins passing through the skin and soft tissues. There is a high risk of infection if the pin sites are not cared for appropriately. The patient should be taught the proper method of pin site cleansing, and to monitor the pins for signs of infection. Any problems should be reported to the surgeon.

Radiography

Radiography is often used during orthopedic surgeries. This technology is particularly useful in the surgical repair and reduction of fractures. The types of radiography most commonly used are the standard x-ray, and fluoroscopy. Fluoroscopy allows the surgeon to view the site of injury as the surgical procedure progresses. It allows the surgeon to confirm that the procedures used in the surgery have been performed correctly, and successfully. The placements of hardware, for example, can be checked while the patient is on the table. The C-arm is a fluoroscopic device that can be positioned directly over the surgical site. Commercial sterile C-arm drapes are available. Fluoroscopes are a type of x-ray, and as such make use of radiation. Depending upon the procedure, the patient may be exposed to relatively high levels of radiation during the use of the fluoroscope.

Tourniquets

Proper Tourniquet Use During Surgery

A tourniquet is used during surgery to reduce blood loss, and to allow a clear view of the surgical field. A tourniquet is usually applied before the extremity in question is prepped and draped. If the surgical site does not allow room for the placement of a non-sterile tourniquet and proper draping of the incision, a sterile tourniquet may be placed after the draping. A tourniquet should be applied snugly with a layer of cast padding between the extremity and the tourniquet. This procedure protects the skin. The full circumference of the involved extremity should be covered by the tourniquet with some overlap at the ends (cuffs) of the tourniquet. Velcro holds the tourniquet in place by securing the tourniquet cuff. If there is a great deal of fatty tissue in the extremity, the tissue should be pulled distally to help place and secure the tourniquet.

Pneumatic Tourniquets

Pneumatic tourniquets are often used during surgeries involving the arms and legs. The tourniquet keeps blood from the surgical site which allows the surgeon a clear view. To start, the blood is pushed out of the area in question by means of elevation, and wrapping. The extremity is wrapped with an ace, or Esmarch, bandage from the distal end to the proximal end. After the area has been drained of blood in this manner, the tourniquet is inflated. The double-cuffed tourniquet is used frequently in surgery, because if 1 cuff does not inflate, the second cuff is sufficient to supply the necessary pressure. Another advantage of the double-cuff tourniquet is that each cuff can be inflated alternately to avoid putting constant pressure on one area. To prevent pressure related damage to the nerves, and blood vessels of the extremity, pressure from the tourniquet should not be applied continuously for more than 1 hour on an arm, or 1 ½ hours on the upper leg.

Methyl Methacrylate

Methyl methacrylate is also called bone cement. This material is customarily used during total joint replacement surgery. Methyl methacrylate stabilizes the implant, and holds it in place. Methyl methacrylate bonds the implant and the bone by filling the spaces in the bone. Methyl methacrylate is freshly mixed for surgery from sterile powder and liquid. The fumes of the mixture are irritating to the mucous membranes, and there is evidence that they are toxic to the liver. There is some evidence as well, that these fumes are damaging to the respiratory tract. For these reasons, the cement is mixed in a closed system with an exhaust device attached to carry away the fumes created by the mixing of the powder, and liquid.

Orthopedic Implants

Orthopedic implants include screws, plates, wires, pins, nails, rods, and joint components. Implants can be manufactured from a number of different alloys. The most common alloys for implants are titanium, stainless steel, and cobalt-chromium. All implants used in a surgery must be made of the same materials. Some alloys may corrode other alloys, and cause the implants to break down. Not only will this delay healing, but may lead to dangerous infection. An implant should not be reused for any reason. Damage to the surface of the implant may cause serious complications including corrosion of the implant, irritation of the bone and other tissues, and infection of the bone and other tissues. For these reasons any implant that has surface damage should not be used. The Food and Drug Administration requires that implants be documented, and traceable.

Sutures

Sutures are used by orthopedic surgeons to hold bone, skin, muscles, blood vessels, ligaments, and tendon together. Sutures must be tough, non-toxic, hypoallergenic, and pliable. Sutures must not carry fluids into the body from outside the body as this could cause infection. There are 2 different types of sutures suitable for different purposes. Absorbable sutures break down in the body over time, and do not require removal. Non-absorbable sutures do not breakdown, and must be manually removed if they cannot be left in indefinitely. The type of suture used depends upon the site of surgery, and the tissue involved. Absorbable sutures are often used internally, and non-absorbable sutures are used externally. This is because of the demands of removal. Non-absorbable sutures, however, are generally used to repair ligaments, tendons, and bone as these tissues have a poor vascular supply, and heal slowly. Absorbable sutures are generally used to close periosteum.

Suture Material

Sutures are made of the following materials: surgical steel, polyester (Ethibond), polypropylene (Prolene), Nylon (Nurolon), chromic, and polyglactin (Vicryl). Each of these materials has different properties. Sutures of different materials are used for different purposes. Surgical steel is the strongest type of suture material, but it lacks elasticity. It is used to join tendons to tendons, and bone to bone. Polyester sutures are braided, and are used to join tendon to bone. Polypropylene sutures are often substituted for stainless steel sutures. This material is easier to handle than stainless steel. It is used to join tendon to bone. Nylon sutures are known to create little tissue reaction. The material is used to join tendon to bone. Chromic sutures are chemically treated to slow absorption. They are used to join periosteum to periosteum. Polyglactin sutures have a slow absorption rate, and are used to join periosteum to periosteum.

Cutting Internal Sutures

The first assistant in surgery cuts the suture for the surgeon after tying. The suture should be cut several millimeters above the knot, leaving a tail. The suture should not be cut too close to the knot, because this could lead to the knot coming untied. If the knot comes untied, the sutured tissue could gape, allowing room for an infection to grow. Conversely, if too long a tail is left this excess suture material could cause a reaction, and could also invite infection. The knot should be approached with the scissors parallel to the tissue. This will ensure that the scissors are perpendicular to the suture. The tips of the scissor blades should be opened to surround the suture. The hand should be supinated 45 degrees before cutting the suture. This will ensure that the knot is not cut, and that the proper length tail remains.

Equipment for Arthroscopic Surgery

Arthroscopy is a minimally invasive surgical procedure used for diagnose purposes, and to repair tissue within a joint. Arthroscopic surgery allows a shorter recovery time than conventional open surgery. Arthroscopies of the knee are a particularly common type of surgery, but this type of surgery is also routinely performed on the ankle, elbow, and wrist joints. The arthroscopic procedure requires a clear view of the interior of the joint. Many types of equipment are required to allow this. The equipment needed includes a video monitor, a light source system, an arthroscopy pump and tubing for fluids, a shaving system with a source of power, a camera, a video recorder, and a system for taking photographs.

Saws, Drills, and Reamers

Orthopedic surgery makes use of instruments powered by air, nitrogen, and electricity. The use of power tools rather than hand-operated tools is more efficient, and makes surgery faster. Power tools have lead to an improvement in surgical technique, and a consequent improvement in postoperative results. The manufacturer provides information regarding the care and cleaning of the power tools, and these instructions must be followed. The surgical assistant should be aware of how the tools to be used work, and should be aware of safety issues. Power saws use one of 2 different motions, and these achieve different effects. The blade of an oscillating saw moves from side to side. The blade of a reciprocating saw moves back and forth. The kind of saw used is dictated by the surgical requirements.

Lasers

The use of lasers in orthopedic surgery is gaining acceptance with improvements in technology and techniques. As technology continues to improve, the use of the laser may continue to increase. The carbon dioxide laser, and Nd:YAG laser are sometimes used during arthroscopies of the knee. These 2 laser types have also been used successfully on soft tissues during total joint arthroplasty, and lumbar laminectomy. The carbon dioxide laser is used to remove methyl methacrylate (bone cement) during a revision arthroplasty. The laser changes the consistency of the methyl methacrylate so that it can be easily separated from the bone. Experimental studies on the possible uses of lasers in orthopedic surgery are now being conducted.

Hemostatic Agents

Hemostatic agents are used to stop bleeding during surgery. Hemostatic agents that are often used in orthopedic surgery include Gelfoam, Avitene, thrombin, and bone wax. Gelfoam comes in a pad form. A piece of this foam is moistened in warm saline, and the excess moisture is squeezed out. The Gelfoam is then applied to the bone at the site where the bleeding is occurring. Avitene is applied dry directly to the bone surface. The produce is applied with forceps, and after application pressure is applied to ensure adhesion. Thrombin is a bovine product that comes in liquid, or powder form. It is available in a spray form. This product must only be used topically. Bone wax is made of sterile beeswax. It is rolled into a ball and applied to the site of bleeding.

Repairing a Syndesmotic Rupture Surgically

A syndesmotic rupture is a tear of the interosseous membrane between the tibia and fibula. Disruption of this membrane allows the two bones to move apart causing instability in the ankle joint. Repair of this injury is necessary to restore normal function. Prior to surgery, the fibula and tibia are moved back into their normal positions, and held in place with a bone clamp. A syndesmotic screw is then inserted distally, under fluoroscopic guidance, to join the fibula to the tibia. Following surgery, the patient must avoid bearing weight on the repaired extremity, or the screw may break. Once the rupture has healed, the screw is removed, and the patient is allowed to resume activities that require weight bearing.

Surgical Dressings

There are a number of reasons surgical dressings are used. They protect the wound from physical damage and from contamination by microbes. They also absorb secretions from the wound. Before a dressing is applied, it must be ensured that the incision site is clean and dry. A skin preparation is applied to the site of the wound. After this, a dressing of suitable size can be applied. The application of a dressing in the operating room is considered part of the surgical procedure, and sterile conditions must be kept. The change of a dressing must also be carried out under sterile conditions. Some types of dressing materials are called dressing sponges. These are not the same as surgical sponges.

One-Layer Dressings

A one-layer dressing is used to dress small wounds with little drainage. This kind of dressing is frequently used to cover areas of intravenous access. A one-layer dressing is made up of a transparent polyurethane film with an adhesive on 1 side. There are many brand name one-layer dressings. These come in many types. Liquid chemical dressings are classified as one-layer dressings. Liquid collodion is one of these. Liquid collodion is applied to the wound and forms a seal over the wound on drying. This product in flammable, however, and may not be permitted in all health care institutes. One-layer dressing types include the following: aerosol adhesive sprays; foams, gels; hydrocolloids; and skin closure tape.

Issues Affecting Choice of Dressing Type

The type of dressing used on a wound depends upon a number of factors. The size of the wound, the type of wound, and the location of the wound affect dressing choice. Some wounds drain more than others and this fact affects dressing choice. The age and size of the patient makes some dressings more appropriate than others. Underlying medical conditions, such as the presence of allergies helps determine the type of dressing chosen. The condition of the skin surrounding the wound makes some dressing types more appropriate. Closed surgical wounds are often dressed with a dry sterile dressing. An antiseptic, or antibiotic, may be used on the wound site before the dressing is applied.

Pressure Dressings and Bulky Dressings

A pressure dressing is a kind of three-layer dressing which is designed to compress the wound. Tissue compression affects the rate of healing. It may help a wound heal more quickly. Too much compression, however, may cause neurovascular compromise and slow the healing process. Pressure dressings may be used for the following reasons: to immobilize the site of the wound; to provide support for the wound; to aid in absorption of fluids; to even out pressure on the wound; to eliminate dead space; to reduce edema; and to reduce hematoma development. The compression in the pressure dressing may result from extra material in the middle layer, or a tightly secured outer layer. A bulky dressing is a three-layer dressing with extra material in the intermediate layer. This extra dressing is designed to immobilize the site, provide support, and absorb fluids.

Three-Layer Dressings

A three-layer dressing is appropriate for wounds that are draining. The three layers of the dressing are as follows: the inner, or contact, layer; the intermediate, or absorbent, layer; and the outer, or securing, layer. These are also called the primary, secondary, and tertiary layers. A three-layer dressing ranges from very simple to extremely complex. A Band-Aid is an example of a simple three-layer dressing. The inner layer can be nonpermeable, semipermeable, or permeable. The intermediate layer covers the inner layer to absorb drainage. The outer layer secures the inner and intermediate layers in position. The outer layer may be made from one of several materials including: tape, wrap, stockinette, tube gauze, or Montgomery straps. Tape is used most frequently.

Specialty Dressings

Specialty dressings have been designed for specific purposes. Examples of specialty dressings include the following: bolster dressing, wet-to-dry dressing, wet-to-wet dressing, thyroid collar, ostomy bag, drain dressing, tracheotomy dressing, eye pad, eye shield, and perineal pad. A bolster dressing is one that is sutured into place. This dressing is also called a stent dressing. It is often used over a graft site to ensure even pressure over the new graft. A wet-to-dry dressing is placed on the site wet, and allowed to dry. This is a form of wound debridement. The dressing is often removed under anesthesia. A wet-to-wet dressing involves the application of a wet dressing which is removed before it is dry. This method provides some wound debridement. A thyroid collar is a neck wrap applied to hold the dressing over a thyroid incision in place. The collar may be commercially made, or made out of a towel.

An ostomy bag is attached over an intestinal stoma to catch secretions. The ostomy bag is attached to the skin by means of an adhesive. A drain dressing is made of gauze sponge. It is shaped to accommodate the drain in a wound. A tracheotomy dressing is positioned around a tracheotomy tube. The tube itself is held in place with umbilical tape tied around the neck. An eye pad is a piece of oval-shaped gauze positioned over the eye to hold medication, and ensure that eye stays closed. An eye shield is an inflexible oval shield positioned over the eye to protect it from pressure. A perineal pad is used to absorb vaginal or perineal fluids.

Rigid Dressing

A rigid dressing is designed to prevent movement, and provide support. Casts and splints are types of rigid dressing. Casts are made of plaster or fiberglass. Splints are generally made of molded plastic, or metal. A splint is applied to 1 surface of a structure. It prevents movement in 1 direction, and provides support. A finger splint, for example may be used to prevent flexion. A cast encases a part of the body. It is applied to prevent movement in any direction, and to provide support. A cast is often applied to immobilize the joints distal and proximal to the injured area. The cylindrical cast is the most common kind of cast. A cast is custom made for the patient.

Transcutaneous Electric Nerve Stimulation

Transcutaneous electric nerve stimulation (TENS) is used to suppress post-operative pain. It does this by stimulating the large-diameter sensory neurons. The TENS unit is portable, and battery operated. The electrodes of the unit are placed directly on the skin near the site of pain. The overstimulation of the target neurons blocks the sensations of pain conducted by unmyelinated nerve fibers. Transcutaneous electric nerve stimulation is often used after total joint replacement surgery, and following the repair of severe fractures. This technology may be used in the control of acute or chronic pain. This technology has the advantages of being non-invasive, non-addictive, and painless. The technology should not be used by individuals with pacemakers, as the electrical current could cause the pacemaker to malfunction.

Continuous Passive Range-of-Motion

Continuous passive range-of-motion, or continuous passive motion (CPM), is used post-operatively to aid recovery from joint surgery. Severe pain is often experienced from joint motion after joint surgery. Because of this, many patients who have had joint surgery avoid moving the joint in question. This can lead to stiffness of the joint, and the formation of scar tissue. CPM is often used to ensure that the patient exercises the joint. CPM can be used while the patient is confined to hospital, or on an outpatient basis. There are CPM machines to treat all the joints of the extremities. CPM uses a machine to start moving the joint gradually. The advantages of CPM are that it can help decrease pain and swelling of the surgical site, improve joint mobility, decrease stiffness of soft tissue, inhibit the formation of adhesions, and prevent muscle wasting.

Electrical Stimulation of Bone

The artificial application of electrical stimulation can increase bone formation. The devices delivering the current come in various types including implantable, percutaneous, and external. A percutaneous stimulator passes the electrical current through the skin. The electrical current generated by these devices is low level. Electrical stimulation is used particularly to treat nonunion, or delayed union. Infected nonunion fractures that have been treated by debridement can also benefit from electrical stimulation, as this helps prevent the growth of bacteria. Electrical stimulation can't be used if there is a large gap between the bone fragments. The disadvantage of using electrical stimulators is that they require the patient to be immobile for an extended period of time. This can delay rehabilitation.

Abduction Slings/Splints Postoperatively for Rotator Cuff Repairs

Rotator cuff tears that cause pain and disability are often treated by surgical repair. The most common technique is to re-attach the torn rotator cuff tendon as close to its natural position as possible on the bone. During repair, the detached tendon can be sutured directly to the bone, or to a secondary anchor. The repaired rotator cuff requires time to rest and heal before being returned to full use. One of the ways to achieve this is abduction splinting. An abduction splint immobilizes the arm so that the humerus is positioned away from the body. This takes tension off of the newly repaired tendon, allowing faster healing, and decreasing the chance of re-injury. These splints are usually comprised of pillow, or pad that is attached to the "body" side of a sling to hold the arm in abduction.

Cervical Halo

A cervical halo is an appliance which immobilizes the head and cervical spine. A cervical halo is comprised of a metal ring fitted around the head, and a vest worn around the chest. These two sections are attached by carbon fiber rods. To begin the application, the metal ring is attached to the patient's head by pins. Each area to be contacted by the pins is thoroughly cleansed, and numbed with a local anesthetic. The two anterior pins at the lateral edge of the forehead are placed near the hairline to minimize scarring. The pins are tightened systemically, and firmly advanced through the scalp into the outer portion of the skull. Once the halo is in place, the vest is put on. The carbon fiber rods are fitted between the metal ring and the vest. These rods are then tightened as needed.

Precautions for Patients with Total Hip Replacement

Total hip replacement surgery involves replacing the acetabulum with an artificial cup, and the femoral head with an artificial head. An artificial joint is created and the artificial acetabulum articulates with the artificial femoral head. The surgery disrupts the tissues surrounding the hip and this can result in the instability of the artificial joint. The patient must to take precautions to help prevent the hip from dislocating. Hip flexion should be limited 90 degrees or less. The patient should avoid sitting in low seats, which could cause an unacceptable level of flexion possibly leading to dislocation. The patient should not cross the legs as this movement could cause sufficient flexion to lever the artificial femoral head out of the acetabulum. Sleeping on the side of the artificial hip should be avoided. To further protect the hip while sleeping, an abduction brace, or several pillows should be positioned between the legs.

OT Practice Test

1. A patient must have a new leg cast applied. When the original cast is removed, the skin surface is covered with scaly, dry, dead skin. The orthopaedic technologist should

a. Gently wash the skin.
b. Brush the skin and apply oil.
c. Lightly brush off dead skin.
d. Leave the skin untouched.

2. A patient in pelvic skin traction is permitted bathroom privileges and asks the orthopaedic technologist to help him get up. The orthopaedic technologist should

a. Remove the weights and leave the pelvic belt in place.
b. Remove the pelvic belt, leaving the weights attached.
c. Remove the weights and then the pelvic belt.
d. Remove the weights and the pelvic belt and apply a back brace.

3. A patient has a splint on the wrist and forearm but has developed window edema between the securing straps. In addition to elevating the extremity, which of the following is the best initial solution?

a. Remove the splint until the edema subsides.
b. Apply wider straps to better distribute the force.
c. Leave the straps loose until the edema subsides.
d. Replace the straps with bias-cut wrapping, from the distal end to the proximal end.

4. A patient is very talkative and, speaking rapidly, gives very long convoluted answers to all questions, making it difficult to obtain an accurate history. The best response for the orthopaedic technologist is to

a. Allow the person to talk freely for five minutes and then interrupt to briefly summarize and clarify the most important points.
b. Tell the person that his/her answers are confusing and they need to be shorter.
c. Allow the person to talk as freely as he/she likes and try to take notes.
d. Ask the patient if a family member can help to provide a history.

5. Which of the following imaging techniques is the most effective for diagnosing osteomyelitis resulting from an infected traumatic injury?

a. Standard radiograph.
b. Computed tomography (CT) scan.
c. Magnetic resonance imaging (MRI).
d. Ultrasound.

6. When assessing a patient's gait, the orthopaedic technologist notes that the patient appears unsteady and uncoordinated with a wide base measurement, and he lifts his feet higher than normal while stepping with the feet flat onto the floor. This gait is characterized as

a. Steppage.
b. Ataxia.
c. Parkinsonian.
d. Scissors.

7. When assessing a patient's level of interest in activities, which of the following information is most essential?

a. Type of activity, past interest, recent past interest, current participation, and future interest in participation.
b. Type of activity and availability of activity resources.
c. Type of activity, cost of activity, and feasibility of participation.
d. Type of activity, physical ability, and current interest.

8. During an interview with an adolescent, the boy ignores the orthopaedic technologist and continues to play a video game on an electronic tablet. The orthopaedic technologist should begin by

a. Telling the boy to put his tablet away.
b. Asking a question and then remaining silent until the boy looks up.
c. Asking the boy if he is feeling anxious about the interview.
d. Asking the boy what kinds of apps he likes.

9. How many major reflexes should the occupational technologist assess when evaluating the musculoskeletal system?

a. Three.
b. Four.
c. Five.
d. Six.

10. A patient is to have side arm skin traction for a fracture of the left humerus. Where are the traction tapes applied?

a. To the upper arm, extending past the elbow and to the forearm, extending to the wrist.
b. To the forearm, extending beyond the hand.
c. To the forearm, extending to the wrist.
d. To the upper arm, extending past the elbow, and to the forearm, extending beyond the hand.

11. A patient must wear a wrist immobilization splint, but the splint tends to migrate as the patient moves her fingers and elbow. Which of the following initial measures is indicated to reduce friction force and migration?

a. Change the size of the splint.
b. Cover her skin with a stockinet or elastic tubular bandage (such as Tubigrip).
c. Increase the number of straps securing the splint.
d. Tighten the straps securing the splint.

12. When applying a cast with extra-fast-setting plaster, the temperature of the water should be

a. Cold.
b. Room temperature.
c. Warm.
d. Hot.

13. When applying cervical skin traction with a head halter, the traction should pull the chin

a. Backward.
b. Upward.
c. Into a neutral position.
d. Down toward the chest.

14. An infant with a clubfoot is receiving progressive plaster casts, and he needs to have the current cast removed. The best method to remove the cast is to

a. Use a cast cutter while he is sleeping.
b. Soak the cast in warm water with 1 tbsp. of vinegar for 1 hour.
c. Soak the cast in warm water with 1 tbsp. vinegar for 10 minutes.
d. Use a cast cutter while the parents hold the child.

15. When the orthopaedic technologist is assessing an elderly patient's functional ability, which test is used specifically to indicate the risk of falls?

a. Katz Activities of Daily Living (ADL) scale.
b. Timed Up and Go (TUG).
c. Functional Ability Rating Scale.
d. Instrumental Activities of Daily Living.

16. When conducting an assessment of the range of motion of the thoracic and lumbar spine, a normal extension when standing is

a. 70 to 90 degrees.
b. 30 to 45 degrees.
c. 20 degrees.
d. 30 degrees.

17. Which of the following is the correct position for the patient during application of a figure-eight clavicle strap for a right clavicular fracture?

a. Sitting in the upright attention position.
b. Leaning forward.
c. Supine.
d. Left-lying.

18. A 30-year-old patient in good physical condition with a non-weight-bearing cast is preparing for discharge. Which method of ambulation is usually indicated?

a. Ambulation with four-wheeled Roll-A-Bout walker.
b. Ambulation with pickup or two-wheeled walker.
c. Crutch walking, three-point gait.
d. Crutch walking, four-point gait.

19. During the initial history to assess a patient for possible arthritis, he complains of stiffness in the knees and hips. The most important follow-up question to aid in diagnosis is

a. "How long does the stiffness persist after a period of inactivity?"
b. "When did the stiffness begin?"
c. "What do you mean when you say 'stiffness'?"
d. "Do you have any skin conditions?"

20. Following total knee replacement, a 50-year-old male's leg is placed in a continuous passive motion (CPM) device with initial settings at 10 degrees extension and 50 degrees flexion. What is the usual extension/flexion goal for discharge?

a. 10 degrees extension, 70 degrees flexion.
b. 0 degrees extension, 90 degrees flexion.
c. 5 degrees extension, 80 degrees flexion.
d. 10 degrees extension and 90 degrees flexion.

21. When conducting the Apley scratch test to assess the rotator cuff, the patient should be instructed to reach with the injured arm and try to

a. Touch the outer rim of the superior medial scapula on the opposite side.
b. Place the hand on the back of the neck.
c. Raise the arm from the side to straight overhead in a half-circle arc.
d. Abduct the arm 90 degrees, and slowly lower the arm.

22. A 70-year-old woman fell on an open and dorsiflexed hand, resulting in a fracture of her distal radius. Two days after closed reduction and application of a short-arm cast, the patient took a shower and got the proximal part of the exterior cast damp. Which initial intervention is indicated?

a. Remove and reapply the cast.
b. Dry the cast with a hair dryer on a cool setting.
c. Allow the cast to air dry only.
d. Replace the cast with a splint.

23. A patient with a long-leg cast complains of pain in the lateral knee area. On examination, the cast is discolored below the knee, and a slight unpleasant odor is present. However, the pulse and circulation in the foot are good. Which of the following complications is most consistent with these signs/symptoms?

a. Compartment syndrome.
b. Pressure ulcer.
c. Fat embolism.
d. Disuse syndrome.

24. The fracture bed position for hip repair places the patient at risk for

a. Sliding and shearing.
b. Back strain.
c. Pressure to genitalia.
d. Diminished lung capacity.

25. When assessing a patient's stride, the orthopaedic technologist would expect an average adult to exhibit about

a. A base width measure of 2 to 4 inches and a 15-inch stride.
b. A base width measure of 1 to 2 inches and a 12-inch stride.
c. A base width measure of 3 to 5 inches and a 20-inch stride.
d. A base width measure of 4 to 6 inches and a 12-inch stride.

26. Which of the following positions is correct for the hamstring muscle test?

a. Sitting.
b. Lateral side-lying.
c. Supine.
d. Prone.

27. When conducting nerve testing of the ulnar nerve for motor function, the orthopaedic technologist asks the patient to

a. Hyperextend the thumb.
b. Touch the tip of the thumb to the tip of the little finger.
c. Abduct all fingers.
d. Adduct all fingers.

28. A patient complains of bouts of recurring pain, erythema, and swelling of the base of the right big toe with sudden onset and symptoms persisting for 3 to 10 days. These symptoms are consistent with

a. Osteoarthritis.
b. Fibromyalgia.
c. Rheumatoid arthritis.
d. Acute gout.

29. When conducting a health history, the four most important areas to assess for a patient with musculoskeletal problems are

a. Pain, comorbidities, swelling, and range of motion.
b. Age, goals, limitations, and pain.
c. Onset of symptoms, degree of pain, age, and range of motion.
d. Onset of symptoms, degree of deformity, paralysis/paresis, and pain.

30. Which of the following imaging techniques is most often used to predict the risk of fractures from osteoporosis?

a. Magnetic resonance imaging (MRI).
b. Computed tomography (CT).
c. Dual-energy x-ray absorptiometry (DXA).
d. Roentgenogram (x-ray).

31. When positioning a supine patient for surgery, the ulnar nerve may be protected by

a. Positioning the arm on an arm board with the palm down (pronated) without further padding.
b. Resting the arm on the trunk with padding under the wrist.
c. Positioning the arm on an arm board with the palm down (pronated) and padding above and below the elbow.
d. Positioning the arm on the table parallel to the body.

32. A leg cast is secure and well fitted, but there is a four-inch stain in the plaster from old bleeding. The best solution to eliminate/cover the stain is to

a. Replace the cast.
b. Cover the stain with white shoe polish.
c. Wipe the stain with a damp cloth.
d. Apply new plaster over the stain.

33. The purpose of separating sponges during surgery is

a. To ensure they are intact.
b. To make counting easier.
c. To facilitate use.
d. To promote better air circulation.

34. During the initial interview and health history, the orthopaedic technologist notes that the patient appears very anxious and is fidgeting, licking her lips, and trembling. The best response for the orthopaedic technologist is

a. "You are trembling. Can you tell me how you are feeling?"
b. "Just relax, I'm only asking questions."
c. "Let's finish this later when you're more relaxed."
d. "Would you like your spouse to answer these questions?"

35. When assessing a patient's short-term memory, which of the following is the best question?

a. "What is your birthdate?"
b. "What was the weather like this morning?"
c. "What did you have for breakfast this morning?"
d. "Can you spell the word WORLD backward?"

36. When assessing a patient for list (lateral tilt of the spine), the orthopaedic technologist should

a. Ask the patient to flex forward at the waist.
b. Draw a line down the spine with a felt-tip pen.
c. Drop a plumb line from T1.
d. Ask the patient to extend backward from the waist.

37. The orthopaedic technologist is changing the dressing of a patient who has had a hip replacement and is experiencing a minimal amount of serosanguineous drainage. Which precautions should the technologist use?

a. Standard.
b. Contact.
c. Standard and contact.
d. Droplet.

38. When bandaging the stump of a patient after an above-the-knee (AK) amputation, the bandaging should start

a. At the base of the stump and be completed by circling the stump horizontally in a superior direction.
b. At the medial anterior surface of the leg and be completed by circling the stump horizontally in an inferior direction.
c. At the base of the stump and be completed with figure-eight turns superiorly.
d. At the medial anterior surface of the leg and be completed with figure-eight turns.

39. After a cast is applied to an arm, the patient should be advised that the drying time for the cast is about

a. 12 hours.
b. 24 hours.
c. 24 to 48 hours.
d. 36 to 72 hours.

40. A patient with a fiberglass long-arm cast has been in a swimming pool and has allowed the cast to get wet, inside and out, believing the lining was waterproof. The fiberglass is dry, but the padding and stockinet remain wet after 24 hours. The best solution is

a. Allow more time for the padding and stockinet to dry.
b. Use a hair dryer to dry the wet material.
c. Replace the cast.
d. Cut wedges in the cast.

41. The type of traction that can include incorporating Kirschner wires or Steinmann pins to a short-arm cast to apply traction on a thumb is

a. Brace traction.
b. Manual traction
c. Skeletal traction
d. Plaster traction.

42. A patient has a fractured femur and is being treated with balanced suspension skeletal traction. What should the orthopaedic technologist do initially when teaching the patient to do quadriceps-setting exercises?

a. Place a hand under the patient's knee.
b. Show the patient a video of the exercise.
c. Review the entire exercise procedure.
d. Tell the patient to tighten the quadriceps muscle.

43. When applying a long-arm cast with the elbow at 90 degrees, the orthopaedic technologist should take extra care to avoid placing too much plaster at the

a. Wrist.
b. Proximal portion of the cast.
c. Elbow flexion crease.
d. Point of the elbow.

44. During the physical examination of a patient, the orthopaedic technologist notes nodules on the dorsolateral aspects of the distal interphalangeal joints (Heberden's nodes). This finding is consistent with

a. Osteoarthritis.
b. Acute rheumatoid arthritis.
c. Chronic rheumatoid arthritis.
d. Trigger finger.

45. When applying a cast to an extremity, padding should be applied

a. From proximal to distal, overlapping each turn by 50%.
b. From distal to proximal, overlapping each turn by 50%.
c. From distal to proximal, using figure-eight turns.
d. From proximal to distal, using figure-eight turns.

46. Following application of a shoulder spica cast, which evaluation by the orthopaedic technologist is most critical?

a. Respiratory status.
b. Blood pressure.
c. Pain level.
d. Neurological status.

47. A thoracolumbosacral orthosis (TLSO) is indicated for treatment of

a. Sprain related to torsion injury.
b. Hyperflexion injury
c. Acute herniated disk.
d. Vertebral fracture.

48. When the orthopaedic technologist is teaching a patient with a non-weight-bearing lower-extremity cast to ascend and descend stairs, the correct instruction for descending is

a. Hop from step to step with the good foot, holding the crutches.
b. Crutches and injured extremity go first and then the well foot.
c. Well foot goes first and then the crutches and injured extremity.
d. Crutches go first and then the well foot and injured extremity.

49. A patient with mild to moderate carpal tunnel syndrome is to be fitted with a splint to wear during the night. The splint should maintain the hand and wrist in which position?

a. Flexion.
b. Extension.
c. Neutral.
d. Varies according to individual needs.

50. An adolescent patient in a one-and-one-half hip spica cast is positioned flat in bed but complains of claustrophobia. Initial measures to alleviate this include

a. Cutting windows in the abdominal area and raising the head of the bed on blocks.
b. Asking the physician for an order for antianxiety medication.
c. Place reflective mirrors so the patient can see forward more easily.
d. Having the patient practice relaxation techniques.

Answer Key and Explanations

1. C: When another cast has to be applied, dead skin should be lightly brushed away, but the skin should not be washed nor oil applied because these will only increase the itching and discomfort when the new cast is applied. If there will not be another cast applied, then the skin should be gently washed and oil should be applied and left on to soften the skin so that the dead skin can be easily washed away in another day or two.

2. B: When removing a patient from pelvic skin traction, the orthopaedic technologist should first remove the weights and then remove the pelvic belt so he doesn't inadvertently trip over the straps. The patient should be advised to keep his back straight and keep his knees higher than his hips when sitting, even on the toilet. Because patients may become lightheaded after prolonged periods of lying down or with pain medications or muscle relaxants, the technologist should assist the patient to walk and then reapply the pelvic belt and weights when he returns to bed.

3. D: To reduce window edema, the straps should be replaced with bias-cut wrapping, applied from the distal end to the proximal end, until the edema subsides because this evens out the distribution of pressure on the skin. The splint should not be removed or the straps loosened so much that the splint is ineffective, leaving the joint unsupported. Wider straps can distribute force better than narrow straps can, but if they are too wide, they may interfere with the range of motion of unimpaired joints.

4. A: Talkative patients can be difficult to interview, so some direction may be necessary; however, often the best approach is to allow the person to talk freely for about five minutes and then gently interrupt to summarize and clarify the main points they've made during the discourse. While the person talks, the orthopaedic technologist should note the patterns of speech and nonverbal behavior as well as the content to determine if the patient appears tense, confused, or psychotic. The technologist should not exhibit impatience or tell the person that his/her answers are confusing.

5. C: Although all of the listed imaging techniques serve a role, the most effective for diagnosis of osteomyelitis is the MRI because it can show the spread of the infection through the bone and the soft tissue. Diagnosis usually begins with standard radiographs to show the overall anatomy and conditions of the bone. Ultrasound is useful for collections of fluid and soft-tissue involvement. CT scans can show the presence of bony abnormalities, but they are not sensitive to osteomyelitis.

6. B: Ataxia: Unsteady and uncoordinated with a wide base measurement and feet lifted higher than normal while stepping with the feet flat onto the floor. Steppage: Dragging or lifting the feet high when walking, then slapping the feet down, giving the appearance of stair walking. Parkinsonian: Walking with the trunk leaning forward with a short, shuffling gait and slight flexion of both hips and knees but without arm swing. Scissors: Thighs crossing while taking short, stiff steps, giving the appearance of someone walking in water.

7. A: Assessment of a patient's level of interest in activities should include the type of activity, past interest (10 years), recent interest (1 year), current participation, and future interest in participation to gain the full picture. Reviewing a checklist of activities with the patient is better than simply asking about activities because recall may be better than production. Activities of interest in the past provide valuable information because sometimes patients stop activities due to disabilities rather than a lack of interest. Current participation and future interests are especially important in planning interventions.

8. D: Asking the boy what kind of apps he likes is a good approach because establishing rapport with an adolescent is often critical to gaining cooperation. A few minutes spent discussing things of interest to the youth is time well spent. The orthopaedic technologist should avoid being confrontational (telling the boy to put his tablet away), and the silent treatment is usually not effective. Adolescents are often self-conscious and resistive to talking about feelings and may be more cooperative if the interview remains less formal.

9. C: Five major reflexes should be assessed when evaluating the musculoskeletal system:

Biceps: Arm flexed at the elbow with the examiner's thumb placed horizontally over biceps tendon with percussion to examiner's thumb.

Brachioradialis: Forearm resting on the leg or the examiner's forearm with percussion to radius at 2 to 5 cm above the wrist.

Triceps: Arm flexed at the elbow with percussion to triceps tendon, about 2 to 5 cm above elbow.

Patellar: Knee bent and leg dangling, with percussion to patellar tendon (directly below the patella).

Achilles tendon: Leg dangling and foot dorsiflexed, percussion to the Achilles tendon right above the heel.

10. D: For side arm skin traction, sets of traction tapes are applied to both the forearm and the upper arm with the upper arm traction tapes extending past the elbow and attached to a spreader and pulley weight equipment to exert a horizontal pull on the humerus. Forearm traction tapes extend beyond the hand and are attached to a spreader and pulley weight equipment to provide a lateral or upward pull and to suspend the arm in a vertical position.

11. B: Some migration is normal with movement because of the friction force between the skin and the splint. Often, covering the skin with a stockinet or elastic tubular bandage (such as Tubigrip) will be sufficient to reduce the friction force that results in movement (kinetic friction). Friction force relates to both the coefficient of fiction (depending on the material) and contact force (the degree of securing and tightening). The friction coefficient of a splint may be increased by lining the splint with foam or applying additional straps, which increases the force of contact.

12. A: Because the warmer the water, the faster the plaster sets, cold water should be used with extra-fast-setting plaster. The roll of plaster should be unrolled so that about two or three inches of plaster extends beyond the roll, and then the roll is immersed in the water until the bubbling stops. The roll is then squeezed and compressed toward the center to remove excess water, taking care not to wring the roll too dry because some of the plaster is lost with the water.

13. D: The purpose of cervical skin traction is to relieve pain, muscle spasms, and neck strain. The traction should pull the chin down toward the chest, flexing the head forward and stretching the muscles at the back of the neck. When applying the head halter, the orthopaedic technologist should gently apply manual traction to ensure that the traction brings the chin into the correct position before applying weights. The patient should lie with the body in proper alignment because body weight and positioning serve as countertraction.

14. B: The best method to remove a cast from an infant or small child is to soak the cast in warm water until the plaster begins to soften and dissolve. The child can be placed in a small tub of warm water with about 1 tbsp. of vinegar added for an hour or so, and then the wrapping can be unrolled and removed. Parents should be advised to do this before the appointment time because using a cast cutter on an infant's cast can cause distress.

15. B: The Timed Up and Go (TUG) test evaluates the time a patient requires to stand from a chair with armrests, walk three meters, turn, return, and sit back down. Those patients requiring ≥14 seconds are at risk for falls. The Katz ADL test evaluates normal activities, such as bathing, dressing, transferring, walking, using the toilet, grooming, and eating and includes timed tests for various activities. Instrumental Activities of Daily Living evaluates ADLs as well as the ability to manage affairs (including finances), arrange transportation, use prosthetic devices, shop, and use the telephone. The Functional Ability Rating Scale evaluates limitations in major life activities, such as self-care, communication, self-direction, the ability to live independently, learning, and the ability to handle economic affairs.

16. D: A normal extension of the thoracic and lumbar spine is 30 degrees when standing and 20 degrees if lying in the prone position. To test for extension with the patient standing, the patient should stand with the feet apart for stability and with the pelvis stabilized and the technologist applying resistance between the patient's scapulae, and then the patient bends backward as far as possible. The range of motion should also include tests for flexion (70 to 90 degrees), lateral movement (35 degrees), and rotation (30 to 45 degrees).

17. A: The patient should sit upright in the attention position for application of the figure-eight clavicle strap because this keeps the bones in proper alignment; however, the patient may require pain medication prior to assuming this position and may need to do so slowly. Prior to application of the strap, the arm and hand on the fracture side should be assessed for neurological or vascular impairment, noting color, temperature, sensation, numbness or tingling, motor function, and strength of pulses.

18. C: A patient in good physical condition with a non-weight-bearing cast is usually instructed in crutch walking with a three-point gait. The four-point gait is used with a partial-weight-bearing cast. Elderly patients and patients with poor balance or an inability to use crutches may use walkers. Two-wheeled or pickup walkers are easy to control, but ambulation is slower because the person must step toward the walker, advance the walker, and then step again. The Roll-A-Bout walker may be used for those who are unable to manage crutches, but it requires weight bearing on the knee.

19. A: Because the stiffness after a period of inactivity is of short duration (such as a few minutes) with degenerative arthritis and tends to persist for a half hour or longer with inflammatory arthritis, including rheumatoid arthritis, "How long does the stiffness persist after a period of inactivity?" is the most important follow-up question. Other questions should include whether the patient also experiences swelling, tenderness, or erythema of joints, has limitations of movement, generalized symptoms (such as chills and fever), or skin conditions (such as a butterfly rash).

20. B: The extension/flexion goal is 0 degrees (full) extension and 90 degrees flexion. The purpose of the CPM device is to promote circulation, decrease the incidence of complications (such as thromboemboli), and increase the range of motion. The CPM device is applied after surgery and should be used as much as possible in the initial postoperative period, although the patient is encouraged to begin ambulation with the knee immobilized and restricted weight bearing within a day of surgery. The leg should be elevated when the patient is sitting.

21. A: Apley's scratch test: The person sits and reaches with the injured arm behind the head and tries to touch the outer rim of the superior medial scapula. Pathology of the rotator cuff (usually the supraspinatus) is indicated by pain or failure to reach the target area. Ludington's sign: The person places both hands behind the neck. A tear is indicated with failure to carry out the action with the affected arm. Drop arm test: The arm is abducted to 90° and slowly lowered. Jerking/dropping indicates tear. Painful arc: The arm is raised in a half-circle arc. Pain between 120 and 170 degrees indicates an injury.

22. B: Drying a cast can be difficult, but the best approach is to use a hair dryer on a cool setting. If the cast is extensively damaged or remains wet on the inside, it may need to be changed to prevent skin irritation or lack of adequate support. A splint is sometimes applied immediately after injury when there is swelling, but it is usually replaced with a cast to ensure that the bones stay in the correct alignment.

23. B: These signs/symptoms are consistent with a pressure ulcer. A window may be cut into the cast or the cast can be bivalved so the area can be examined and treated. Compartment syndrome is characterized by impaired circulation and is treated by bivalving the cast and elevating the limb. If symptoms persist, a fasciotomy is needed. A fat embolism results in systemic effects, such as hypoxia, tachypnea, fever, and tachycardia, and it is an emergent condition. Disuse syndrome results in atrophy and weakness of muscles and is prevented by muscle-setting exercises (such as quadriceps and gluteal setting).

24. C: The fracture bed position, used for hip fracture repair or closed nailing of the femur, places the patient at an increased risk for pressure on the genitalia and pressure in the foot and ankle in traction. The patient is in the supine position with a perineal post to stabilize the pelvis. The perineal post must be adequately padded, and the position of genitals, especially for a male, must be checked for compression because pressure may cause damage. Additionally, pressure on the perineal area can result in damage to the perineal and pudendal nerves.

25. A: Although gaits vary, the average base width measure, the distance between the patient's heels as they pass each other when he or she walks, is 2 to 4 inches with a 15-inch stride. The technologist should begin the assessment when the patient is unaware, such as when the patient enters a room, because people may alter their gait when they are aware of being assessed. The patient's posture, rhythm, balance, and arm swings should also be assessed. As the patient turns, the face and head should precede the rest of the body.

26. D: Hamstring muscle test: The patient lies in the prone position, and the technologist places one hand on the thigh to stabilize it. Then, the patient flexes the knee, elevating the foot and extending the leg against resistance. Quadriceps muscle test: The patient sits with his or her leg dangling, and the technologist places one hand on the thigh to stabilize it while the patient attempts to extend and straighten the leg against resistance.

27. C: Ulnar nerve: Ask the patient to abduct all fingers, spreading them open. Additional testing includes pricking the distal fad pad of the little finger. Radial nerve: Ask the patient to hyperextend the thumb or wrist (creating an L-shape between the thumb and index finger). Additional testing includes pricking the webbing between the thumb and index finger. Median nerve: Ask the patient to touch the tip of the thumb to the tip of the little finger. Additional testing includes pricking the distal surface of the index finger.

28. D: Gout (metabolic arthritis) is a group of conditions associated with a defect of purine metabolism that results in hyperuricemia with oversecretion of uric acid, decreased excretion of uric acid, or a combination. The increased uric acid levels can cause monosodium urate crystal depositions in the joints, resulting in severe articular and periarticular inflammation. Symptoms include abrupt onset of pain with erythema and edema lasting 3 to 10 days, usually involving one joint, such as the base of the big toe, in the beginning episodes.

29. D: Onset of symptoms: Note how and when the symptoms started and any contributing factors, including a review of treatments. Degree of deformity: Evaluate pain, swelling, stiffness, and reports of limitations. Observe for changes such as enlarged joints. Paralysis/paresis: Note the onset and extent and any changes such as regression or progression of symptoms. Pain: Note the type of pain, where it's located, the severity, duration, any contributing or precipitating factors, and any other symptoms associated with the pain (such as increased weakness).

30. C: Dual-energy x-ray absorptiometry (DXA) scans are the gold standard for determining the degree of osteoporosis and predicting the risk of fractures with vertebral fractures followed by hip fractures, the most common fractures in postmenopausal woman. Results of bone mineral density are expressed as T-scores:

T-score:	Bone Mass:
0 to 1.0	Normal
-1.0	10% below normal
-2.0	20% below normal (osteoporosis)

31. C: The ulnar nerve may be protected in a number of ways:

- Positioning the arm on an arm board with the palm down (pronated) and padding above and below the elbow.
- Positioning the arm on an arm board with the palm up (supinated).
- Positioning the arm across the chest with padding under the upper arm.

Arms should not be positioned alongside the body unless absolutely necessary because they may slip out of place during surgery or lie against the edge of the bed. The arms should be secured by a draw sheet, using care to avoid pressure or tight folds across the elbow.

32. D: The best solution to eliminate a fairly large stain on a cast is to apply new plaster over the stain in a thin layer. Once this dries, the stain will no longer be evident. Patients should be advised to take care to avoid soiling a cast, but small stains can be covered with white shoe polish, and the cast can be wiped with a damp (NOT wet) cloth to remove surface dirt. Patients should be advised to cover casts with clothing as much as possible.

33. B: Sponges should be separated and counted out loud during the initial count to ensure that the count is accurate and that each package contains the correct number of sponges. The circulating nurse and one other person should participate in the count. Used sponges should also be kept separated for counting. If a package holds an incorrect number, the entire package should be removed, bagged, labeled, and isolated from the sterile field. The same sequence of counting (large to small, small to large, or proximal to distal) should be used during every count because an established routine minimizes errors.

34. A: "You are trembling. Can you tell me how you are feeling?" is the best response because it acknowledges what the technologist sees and encourages the patient to express feelings. Many people become quite nervous when interviewed, and stress may be contributing to their illness. Nonverbal clues, such as fidgeting, licking the lips, rubbing the hands together, or trembling, may indicate anxiety. Some people talk rapidly and nervously when anxious, whereas others remain silent and withdrawn.

35. B: "What was the weather like this morning?" tests short-term memory with a question whose answer the orthopaedic technologist can verify from personal experience. Patients may sometimes make up answers to questions such as "What did you have for breakfast this morning?" to cover their memory loss. Tasks such as spelling words backward are used to test attention, and asking questions about past events, such as the person's birthdate, tests long-term memory.

36. C: To assess for list (lateral tilt of the spine), the orthopaedic technologist should drop a plumb line from T1 (spinous process) and check to see where the line falls. A list is evident if the plumb line falls to one side of the gluteal cleft rather than midline. A list occurs with scoliosis, which is best observed by asking the patient to flex forward. If the body compensates for the curvature of scoliosis, then a plumb line dropped from T1 lands midline.

37. A: The orthopaedic technologist should use standard precautions, which are indicated for all patients and all contact with bodily fluids, such as urine, feces, and serous and sanguineous drainage. This should include hand hygiene, gloves, and gown while changing the dressing. Contact precautions are indicated for draining or infected wounds and require the use of gowns and gloves for all contact with the patient or the immediate patient environment to prevent the spread of an infection from one patient to another.

38. D: The purpose of bandaging an above-the-knee (AK) amputation is to help to control edema and shape the stump so that a prosthesis can be fitted. The bandaging should be done using a long roll of four-inch elastic bandage with wrapping beginning at the medial anterior surface of the leg (near the groin), using figure-eight turns to gradually apply increasing pressure from the base of the stump superiorly. The bandage should not encircle the stump horizontally because this may cause decreased circulation.

39. B: A standard cast on an arm or leg usually dries in about 24 hours, whereas weight-bearing casts can require 24 to 48 hours to dry. Larger body casts can require 36 to 72 hours to dry thoroughly. When dry, the plaster of Paris should appear very white and shiny, and it should be free of odor. The orthopaedic technologist can check the cast by tapping on it to elicit a resonant sound. Some types of fast-setting plaster may dry more quickly.

40. C: In this case, the best solution is to replace the cast because it may be impossible to adequately circulate enough warm air through the cast to dry the padding and stockinet, and even small areas of dampness may result in maceration of the skin. When the cast is removed, the skin should be carefully examined before application of a new cast because the skin can become damaged very rapidly, especially if the dampness caused the padding to wad up and apply pressure.

41. D: Plaster traction: Including Kirschner wires or Steinmann pins in a cast to provide a continuous pulling force. Brace traction: Using a brace to exert traction, such as with hyperextension braces. Manual traction: Using hands to apply direct traction, as with reducing dislocations. It may be used when mechanical traction is released and readjusted and while someone is applying a cast to maintain alignment. Skeletal traction: Applying traction directly to the skeletal system through the use of tongs, pins, screws, or wires.

42. A: Patients with skeletal traction to a lower extremity should exercise regularly to prevent muscle weakness and contractures. The best way to begin quadriceps-setting exercises is for the orthopaedic technologist to place one hand under the patient's knee and ask the patient to tighten the quadriceps muscle and press down on the hand. Patients are often very guarded in using joints because of the fear of pain, so placing a hand under the knee is reassuring and also allows the technologist to feel the patient contracting the muscles. The patient should hold for a count of 5 and then relax for a count of 5, gradually repeating up to 20 times.

43. C: The orthopaedic technologist should take extra care to avoid placing excessive plaster in the flexion crease of the elbow because this can interfere with circulation, which may already be somewhat compromised by the 90-degree positioning. The cast should be trimmed around the knuckles and across the proximal flexion crease on the palm side so that the fingers can move freely, making sure there are no sharp edges that might irritate the skin.

44. A: Osteoarthritis: Heberden's nodes on the distal interphalangeal joints are common. Bouchard's nodes on the proximal interphalangeal joints may also occur. Acute rheumatoid arthritis: Joints become painful, swollen, and stiff, but the distal interphalangeal joints are rarely affected. Chronic rheumatoid arthritis: Fingers develop a "swan-neck" deformity (hyperextension of the proximal interphalangeal joints with fixed flexion of the distal interphalangeal joints) and boutonniere deformity (flexion of the proximal interphalangeal joint with hyperextension of the distal interphalangeal joint). Trigger finger: Fingers "catch" in the flexed position and snap into extension because of a nodule in the flexor tendon in the palm.

45. B: Padding is applied from the distal end to the proximal end, overlapping each turn by 50%. A stockinet may be applied under the padding, but it is often applied only at the upper and lower ends because it may cause tension over bony prominences and result in pain or pressure sores. Padding is usually four to six inches wide for a lower extremity casting and two to four inches wide for an upper extremity casting. An extra layer of padding is sometimes added over bony prominences, especially in very slender patients, although excessive padding should be avoided because it may clump or prevent a tight fit of the cast.

46. A: Although all of these are important, because the shoulder spica cast encases the chest, the patient's respiratory status must be assessed first because if the patient cannot breathe adequately, he or she may become hypoxic. The rate, depth, and rhythm of breathing should all be assessed by asking the patient to take deep breaths and carefully observing his or her response, including color. Patients may be quite stressed and may feel short of breath because of the restriction of the cast even if they are breathing adequately. The patient should be carefully aligned and supported with pillows.

47. A: A thoracolumbosacral orthosis (TLSO) is indicated for treatment of torsion injuries caused by twisting and sprain. These are the most common lower back injuries, usually at L4 to L5. The usual treatment is a few days of bed rest and then resumption of activities while wearing the brace to prevent twisting or hyperextension, which may result in chronic injury and pain. Torsion injuries tend to heal slowly, so patients should be advised of the need to continue to wear the brace until they are well healed.

48. D: Descending: Crutches go first and then the well foot and the injured extremity. Ascending: Well foot goes first and then crutches and the injured extremity.

The patient should be cautioned not to bear weight under the axillae because this can cause nerve damage but, rather, to hold the crutches tightly against the side of the chest wall. Typical gaits include:

- Two-point, in which both crutches are placed forward and then the well leg advances to the crutches.
- Three-point, in which the injured extremity and both crutches are advanced together and then the well leg advances to the crutches.

49. C: Carpal tunnel syndrome occurs when the median nerve is compressed in the carpal tunnel, resulting in paresthesia with pain and numbness along the nerve distribution. Mild to moderate carpal tunnel syndrome may be alleviated by wearing a splint either during the night only or full time. The splint holds the wrist and hand in a neutral position to prevent hyperextension or extended flexion because these positions can cause further compression of the nerve. More severe symptoms may require surgical intervention.

50. A: The initial measures to relieve the claustrophobia that some patients experience with hip spica casts are to cut windows in the abdominal area of the cast so that the patient feels less constricted and to raise the head of the bed on four- or eight-inch blocks because some patients experience the feeling that their heads are below their trunks and, because their range of vision is limited, this adds to their feelings of claustrophobia. Relaxation techniques may also be of some value.

How to Overcome Test Anxiety

Just the thought of taking a test is enough to make most people a little nervous. A test is an important event that can have a long-term impact on your future, so it's important to take it seriously and it's natural to feel anxious about performing well. But just because anxiety is normal, that doesn't mean that it's helpful in test taking, or that you should simply accept it as part of your life. Anxiety can have a variety of effects. These effects can be mild, like making you feel slightly nervous, or severe, like blocking your ability to focus or remember even a simple detail.

If you experience test anxiety—whether severe or mild—it's important to know how to beat it. To discover this, first you need to understand what causes test anxiety.

Causes of Test Anxiety

While we often think of anxiety as an uncontrollable emotional state, it can actually be caused by simple, practical things. One of the most common causes of test anxiety is that a person does not feel adequately prepared for their test. This feeling can be the result of many different issues such as poor study habits or lack of organization, but the most common culprit is time management. Starting to study too late, failing to organize your study time to cover all of the material, or being distracted while you study will mean that you're not well prepared for the test. This may lead to cramming the night before, which will cause you to be physically and mentally exhausted for the test. Poor time management also contributes to feelings of stress, fear, and hopelessness as you realize you are not well prepared but don't know what to do about it.

Other times, test anxiety is not related to your preparation for the test but comes from unresolved fear. This may be a past failure on a test, or poor performance on tests in general. It may come from comparing yourself to others who seem to be performing better or from the stress of living up to expectations. Anxiety may be driven by fears of the future—how failure on this test would affect your educational and career goals. These fears are often completely irrational, but they can still negatively impact your test performance.

Review Video: 3 Reasons You Have Test Anxiety
Visit mometrix.com/academy and enter code: 428468

Elements of Test Anxiety

As mentioned earlier, test anxiety is considered to be an emotional state, but it has physical and mental components as well. Sometimes you may not even realize that you are suffering from test anxiety until you notice the physical symptoms. These can include trembling hands, rapid heartbeat, sweating, nausea, and tense muscles. Extreme anxiety may lead to fainting or vomiting. Obviously, any of these symptoms can have a negative impact on testing. It is important to recognize them as soon as they begin to occur so that you can address the problem before it damages your performance.

Review Video: 3 Ways to Tell You Have Test Anxiety
Visit mometrix.com/academy and enter code: 927847

The mental components of test anxiety include trouble focusing and inability to remember learned information. During a test, your mind is on high alert, which can help you recall information and stay focused for an extended period of time. However, anxiety interferes with your mind's natural processes, causing you to blank out, even on the questions you know well. The strain of testing during anxiety makes it difficult to stay focused, especially on a test that may take several hours. Extreme anxiety can take a huge mental toll, making it difficult not only to recall test information but even to understand the test questions or pull your thoughts together.

Review Video: How Test Anxiety Affects Memory
Visit mometrix.com/academy and enter code: 609003

Effects of Test Anxiety

Test anxiety is like a disease—if left untreated, it will get progressively worse. Anxiety leads to poor performance, and this reinforces the feelings of fear and failure, which in turn lead to poor performances on subsequent tests. It can grow from a mild nervousness to a crippling condition. If allowed to progress, test anxiety can have a big impact on your schooling, and consequently on your future.

Test anxiety can spread to other parts of your life. Anxiety on tests can become anxiety in any stressful situation, and blanking on a test can turn into panicking in a job situation. But fortunately, you don't have to let anxiety rule your testing and determine your grades. There are a number of relatively simple steps you can take to move past anxiety and function normally on a test and in the rest of life.

Review Video: How Test Anxiety Impacts Your Grades
Visit mometrix.com/academy and enter code: 939819

Physical Steps for Beating Test Anxiety

While test anxiety is a serious problem, the good news is that it can be overcome. It doesn't have to control your ability to think and remember information. While it may take time, you can begin taking steps today to beat anxiety.

Just as your first hint that you may be struggling with anxiety comes from the physical symptoms, the first step to treating it is also physical. Rest is crucial for having a clear, strong mind. If you are tired, it is much easier to give in to anxiety. But if you establish good sleep habits, your body and mind will be ready to perform optimally, without the strain of exhaustion. Additionally, sleeping well helps you to retain information better, so you're more likely to recall the answers when you see the test questions.

Getting good sleep means more than going to bed on time. It's important to allow your brain time to relax. Take study breaks from time to time so it doesn't get overworked, and don't study right before bed. Take time to rest your mind before trying to rest your body, or you may find it difficult to fall asleep.

Review Video: The Importance of Sleep for Your Brain
Visit mometrix.com/academy and enter code: 319338

Along with sleep, other aspects of physical health are important in preparing for a test. Good nutrition is vital for good brain function. Sugary foods and drinks may give a burst of energy but this burst is followed by a crash, both physically and emotionally. Instead, fuel your body with protein and vitamin-rich foods.

Also, drink plenty of water. Dehydration can lead to headaches and exhaustion, especially if your brain is already under stress from the rigors of the test. Particularly if your test is a long one, drink water during the breaks. And if possible, take an energy-boosting snack to eat between sections.

Review Video: How Diet Can Affect your Mood
Visit mometrix.com/academy and enter code: 624317

Along with sleep and diet, a third important part of physical health is exercise. Maintaining a steady workout schedule is helpful, but even taking 5-minute study breaks to walk can help get your blood pumping faster and clear your head. Exercise also releases endorphins, which contribute to a positive feeling and can help combat test anxiety.

When you nurture your physical health, you are also contributing to your mental health. If your body is healthy, your mind is much more likely to be healthy as well. So take time to rest, nourish your body with healthy food and water, and get moving as much as possible. Taking these physical steps will make you stronger and more able to take the mental steps necessary to overcome test anxiety.

Review Video: How to Stay Healthy and Prevent Test Anxiety
Visit mometrix.com/academy and enter code: 877894

Mental Steps for Beating Test Anxiety

Working on the mental side of test anxiety can be more challenging, but as with the physical side, there are clear steps you can take to overcome it. As mentioned earlier, test anxiety often stems from lack of preparation, so the obvious solution is to prepare for the test. Effective studying may be the most important weapon you have for beating test anxiety, but you can and should employ several other mental tools to combat fear.

First, boost your confidence by reminding yourself of past success—tests or projects that you aced. If you're putting as much effort into preparing for this test as you did for those, there's no reason you should expect to fail here. Work hard to prepare; then trust your preparation.

Second, surround yourself with encouraging people. It can be helpful to find a study group, but be sure that the people you're around will encourage a positive attitude. If you spend time with others who are anxious or cynical, this will only contribute to your own anxiety. Look for others who are motivated to study hard from a desire to succeed, not from a fear of failure.

Third, reward yourself. A test is physically and mentally tiring, even without anxiety, and it can be helpful to have something to look forward to. Plan an activity following the test, regardless of the outcome, such as going to a movie or getting ice cream.

When you are taking the test, if you find yourself beginning to feel anxious, remind yourself that you know the material. Visualize successfully completing the test. Then take a few deep, relaxing breaths and return to it. Work through the questions carefully but with confidence, knowing that you are capable of succeeding.

Developing a healthy mental approach to test taking will also aid in other areas of life. Test anxiety affects more than just the actual test—it can be damaging to your mental health and even contribute to depression. It's important to beat test anxiety before it becomes a problem for more than testing.

Review Video: Test Anxiety and Depression
Visit mometrix.com/academy and enter code: 904704

Study Strategy

Being prepared for the test is necessary to combat anxiety, but what does being prepared look like? You may study for hours on end and still not feel prepared. What you need is a strategy for test prep. The next few pages outline our recommended steps to help you plan out and conquer the challenge of preparation.

Step 1: Scope Out the Test

Learn everything you can about the format (multiple choice, essay, etc.) and what will be on the test. Gather any study materials, course outlines, or sample exams that may be available. Not only will this help you to prepare, but knowing what to expect can help to alleviate test anxiety.

Step 2: Map Out the Material

Look through the textbook or study guide and make note of how many chapters or sections it has. Then divide these over the time you have. For example, if a book has 15 chapters and you have five days to study, you need to cover three chapters each day. Even better, if you have the time, leave an extra day at the end for overall review after you have gone through the material in depth.

If time is limited, you may need to prioritize the material. Look through it and make note of which sections you think you already have a good grasp on, and which need review. While you are studying, skim quickly through the familiar sections and take more time on the challenging parts. Write out your plan so you don't get lost as you go. Having a written plan also helps you feel more in control of the study, so anxiety is less likely to arise from feeling overwhelmed at the amount to cover.

Step 3: Gather Your Tools

Decide what study method works best for you. Do you prefer to highlight in the book as you study and then go back over the highlighted portions? Or do you type out notes of the important information? Or is it helpful to make flashcards that you can carry with you? Assemble the pens, index cards, highlighters, post-it notes, and any other materials you may need so you won't be distracted by getting up to find things while you study.

If you're having a hard time retaining the information or organizing your notes, experiment with different methods. For example, try color-coding by subject with colored pens, highlighters, or post-it notes. If you learn better by hearing, try recording yourself reading your notes so you can listen while in the car, working out, or simply sitting at your desk. Ask a friend to quiz you from your flashcards, or try teaching someone the material to solidify it in your mind.

Step 4: Create Your Environment

It's important to avoid distractions while you study. This includes both the obvious distractions like visitors and the subtle distractions like an uncomfortable chair (or a too-comfortable couch that makes you want to fall asleep). Set up the best study environment possible: good lighting and a comfortable work area. If background music helps you focus, you may want to turn it on, but otherwise keep the room quiet. If you are using a computer to take notes, be sure you don't have any other windows open, especially applications like social media, games, or anything else that could distract you. Silence your phone and turn off notifications. Be sure to keep water close by so you stay hydrated while you study (but avoid unhealthy drinks and snacks).

Also, take into account the best time of day to study. Are you freshest first thing in the morning? Try to set aside some time then to work through the material. Is your mind clearer in the afternoon or evening? Schedule your study session then. Another method is to study at the same time of day that you will take the test, so that your brain gets used to working on the material at that time and will be ready to focus at test time.

Step 5: Study!

Once you have done all the study preparation, it's time to settle into the actual studying. Sit down, take a few moments to settle your mind so you can focus, and begin to follow your study plan. Don't give in to distractions or let yourself procrastinate. This is your time to prepare so you'll be ready to fearlessly approach the test. Make the most of the time and stay focused.

Of course, you don't want to burn out. If you study too long you may find that you're not retaining the information very well. Take regular study breaks. For example, taking five minutes out of every hour to walk briskly, breathing deeply and swinging your arms, can help your mind stay fresh.

As you get to the end of each chapter or section, it's a good idea to do a quick review. Remind yourself of what you learned and work on any difficult parts. When you feel that you've mastered the material, move on to the next part. At the end of your study session, briefly skim through your notes again.

But while review is helpful, cramming last minute is NOT. If at all possible, work ahead so that you won't need to fit all your study into the last day. Cramming overloads your brain with more information than it can process and retain, and your tired mind may struggle to recall even previously learned information when it is overwhelmed with last-minute study. Also, the urgent nature of cramming and the stress placed on your brain contribute to anxiety. You'll be more likely to go to the test feeling unprepared and having trouble thinking clearly.

So don't cram, and don't stay up late before the test, even just to review your notes at a leisurely pace. Your brain needs rest more than it needs to go over the information again. In fact, plan to finish your studies by noon or early afternoon the day before the test. Give your brain the rest of the day to relax or focus on other things, and get a good night's sleep. Then you will be fresh for the test and better able to recall what you've studied.

Step 6: Take a practice test

Many courses offer sample tests, either online or in the study materials. This is an excellent resource to check whether you have mastered the material, as well as to prepare for the test format and environment.

Check the test format ahead of time: the number of questions, the type (multiple choice, free response, etc.), and the time limit. Then create a plan for working through them. For example, if you have 30 minutes to take a 60-question test, your limit is 30 seconds per question. Spend less time on the questions you know well so that you can take more time on the difficult ones.

If you have time to take several practice tests, take the first one open book, with no time limit. Work through the questions at your own pace and make sure you fully understand them. Gradually work up to taking a test under test conditions: sit at a desk with all study materials put away and set a timer. Pace yourself to make sure you finish the test with time to spare and go back to check your answers if you have time.

After each test, check your answers. On the questions you missed, be sure you understand why you missed them. Did you misread the question (tests can use tricky wording)? Did you forget the information? Or was it something you hadn't learned? Go back and study any shaky areas that the practice tests reveal.

Taking these tests not only helps with your grade, but also aids in combating test anxiety. If you're already used to the test conditions, you're less likely to worry about it, and working through tests until you're scoring well gives you a confidence boost. Go through the practice tests until you feel comfortable, and then you can go into the test knowing that you're ready for it.

Test Tips

On test day, you should be confident, knowing that you've prepared well and are ready to answer the questions. But aside from preparation, there are several test day strategies you can employ to maximize your performance.

First, as stated before, get a good night's sleep the night before the test (and for several nights before that, if possible). Go into the test with a fresh, alert mind rather than staying up late to study.

Try not to change too much about your normal routine on the day of the test. It's important to eat a nutritious breakfast, but if you normally don't eat breakfast at all, consider eating just a protein bar. If you're a coffee drinker, go ahead and have your normal coffee. Just make sure you time it so that the caffeine doesn't wear off right in the middle of your test. Avoid sugary beverages, and drink enough water to stay hydrated but not so much that you need a restroom break 10 minutes into the test. If your test isn't first thing in the morning, consider going for a walk or doing a light workout before the test to get your blood flowing.

Allow yourself enough time to get ready, and leave for the test with plenty of time to spare so you won't have the anxiety of scrambling to arrive in time. Another reason to be early is to select a good seat. It's helpful to sit away from doors and windows, which can be distracting. Find a good seat, get out your supplies, and settle your mind before the test begins.

When the test begins, start by going over the instructions carefully, even if you already know what to expect. Make sure you avoid any careless mistakes by following the directions.

Then begin working through the questions, pacing yourself as you've practiced. If you're not sure on an answer, don't spend too much time on it, and don't let it shake your confidence. Either skip it and come back later, or eliminate as many wrong answers as possible and guess among the remaining ones. Don't dwell on these questions as you continue—put them out of your mind and focus on what lies ahead.

Be sure to read all of the answer choices, even if you're sure the first one is the right answer. Sometimes you'll find a better one if you keep reading. But don't second-guess yourself if you do immediately know the answer. Your gut instinct is usually right. Don't let test anxiety rob you of the information you know.

If you have time at the end of the test (and if the test format allows), go back and review your answers. Be cautious about changing any, since your first instinct tends to be correct, but make sure you didn't misread any of the questions or accidentally mark the wrong answer choice. Look over any you skipped and make an educated guess.

At the end, leave the test feeling confident. You've done your best, so don't waste time worrying about your performance or wishing you could change anything. Instead, celebrate the successful completion of this test. And finally, use this test to learn how to deal with anxiety even better next time.

Review Video: 5 Tips to Beat Test Anxiety
Visit mometrix.com/academy and enter code: 570656

Important Qualification

Not all anxiety is created equal. If your test anxiety is causing major issues in your life beyond the classroom or testing center, or if you are experiencing troubling physical symptoms related to your anxiety, it may be a sign of a serious physiological or psychological condition. If this sounds like your situation, we strongly encourage you to seek professional help.

Thank You

We at Mometrix would like to extend our heartfelt thanks to you, our friend and patron, for allowing us to play a part in your journey. It is a privilege to serve people from all walks of life who are unified in their commitment to building the best future they can for themselves.

The preparation you devote to these important testing milestones may be the most valuable educational opportunity you have for making a real difference in your life. We encourage you to put your heart into it—that feeling of succeeding, overcoming, and yes, conquering will be well worth the hours you've invested.

We want to hear your story, your struggles and your successes, and if you see any opportunities for us to improve our materials so we can help others even more effectively in the future, please share that with us as well. **The team at Mometrix would be absolutely thrilled to hear from you!** So please, send us an email (support@mometrix.com) and let's stay in touch.

If you'd like some additional help, check out these other resources we offer for your exam:
http://MometrixFlashcards.com/OrthopaedicTech

Additional Bonus Material

Due to our efforts to try to keep this book to a manageable length, we've created a link that will give you access to all of your additional bonus material.

Please visit https://www.mometrix.com/bonus948/orthtech to access the information.